Register Now for Online Access to Your Book!

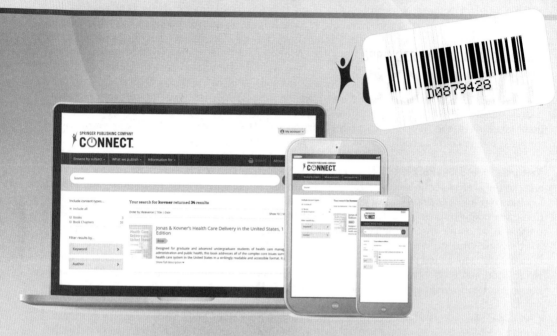

Wanda E. Bonnel, PhD, APRN, ANEF, is an associate professor at the University of Kansas School of Nursing, Kansas City, Kansas. As a specialist in geriatrics and nursing education, she teaches courses in the master's, Doctor of Nursing Practice (DNP), and doctoral programs. She is a fellow in the National League for Nursing Academy of Nursing Education and recipient of the Chancellor's Distinguished Teaching Award at the University of Kansas. Dr. Bonnel has received multiple funded grants, including the Health Resources & Services Administration (HRSA) online Health Professions Educator Certificate program. She has published numerous peer-reviewed abstracts and articles in educator and geriatric specialty journals. She has also coauthored the textbook *Proposal Writing for Clinical Nursing and DNP Projects* (2017). Her ongoing research interests include online learning, best practices, and advanced practice mentoring. Dr. Bonnel has served as grant reviewer for the National League for Nursing and HRSA, a manuscript reviewer for multiple journals, and an editorial board member of the *Journal of Gerontological Nursing*.

Katharine Vogel Smith, PhD, RN, CNE, is an associate professor and assistant dean for program evaluation at the University of Missouri–Kansas City School of Nursing and Health Studies. Dr. Smith has received multiple grants, most of which have focused on aspects of teaching, advanced education, and nursing traineeships. Recent scholarship includes peer-reviewed publications and national presentations on the use of simulation to teach legal and ethical content. She has also coauthored the textbook *Proposal Writing for Clinical Nursing and DNP Projects* (2017). Dr. Smith teaches in both undergraduate and graduate nursing programs, facilitating advanced clinical projects through the institutional review board process. She also conducts program review and site visits for both nursing and non-nursing programs and serves as a manuscript reviewer for selected journals.

Christine L. Hober, PhD, RN-BC, CNE, is a professor at Fort Hays State University, Hays, Kansas. A PhD graduate from the University of Kansas, she brings years of diverse experiences in teaching and administration in a rural nursing program. She maintains National Certification in both Medical-Surgical Nursing and Nursing Education. She brings experience from the education committee of the Kansas State Board of Nursing. Dr. Hober has completed multiple research projects on simulation. She has presented and published her work on teaching and learning best practices in multiple venues.

SECOND EDITION

Teaching With Technologies in Nursing and the Health Professions

Strategies for Engagement, Quality, and Safety

WANDA E. BONNEL, PhD, APRN, ANEF

KATHARINE VOGEL SMITH, PhD, RN, CNE

CHRISTINE L. HOBER, PhD, RN-BC, CNE

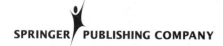
SPRINGER PUBLISHING COMPANY

Springer Publishing Company, LLC
11 West 42nd Street
New York, NY 10036
www.springerpub.com

Acquisitions Editor: Joseph Morita
Managing Editor: Cindy Yoo
Compositor: Graphic World

ISBN: 978-0-8261-4279-5
ebook ISBN: 978-0-8261-4292-4

Instructor's Materials: Qualified instructors may request supplements by emailing textbook@springerpub.com:
Instructor's Manual: 978-0-8261-4253-5
Instructor's PowerPoints: 978-0-8261-4246-7

18 19 20 21 22 5 4 3 2 1

The author and the publisher of this Work have made every effort to use sources believed to be reliable to provide information that is accurate and compatible with the standards generally accepted at the time of publication. The author and publisher shall not be liable for any special, consequential, or exemplary damages resulting, in whole or in part, from the readers' use of, or reliance on, the information contained in this book. The publisher has no responsibility for the persistence or accuracy of URLs for external or third-party Internet websites referred to in this publication and does not guarantee that any content on such websites is, or will remain, accurate or appropriate.

Library of Congress Cataloging-in-Publication Data

Names: Bonnel, Wanda E., editor. | Smith, Katharine Vogel, editor. | Hober,
    Christine L., editor.
Title: Teaching with technologies in nursing and the health professions :
    strategies for engagement, quality, and safety / [edited by] Wanda E.
    Bonnel, Katharine V. Smith, Christine L. Hober.
Other titles: Teaching technologies in nursing and the health professions
Description: Second edition. | New York, NY : Springer Publishing Company,
    LLC, [2019] | Preceded by Teaching technologies in nursing and the health
    professions / [edited by] Wanda E. Bonnel, Katharine Vogel Smith. 2010. |
    Includes bibliographical references and index.
Identifiers: LCCN 2018009644 (print) | LCCN 2018010512 (ebook) | ISBN
    9780826142795 | ISBN 9780826142795 (pbk.) | ISBN 9780826142924 (ebook)
    | ISBN 9780826142535 (instructors manual) | ISBN 9780826142467
    (instructors PowerPoints)
Subjects: | MESH: Education, Nursing—methods | Computer-Assisted
    Instruction—methods | Internet | Education, Nursing, Continuing—trends |
    Educational Technology—trends
Classification: LCC RT71 (ebook) | LCC RT71 (print) | NLM WY 18 | DDC
    610.73076—dc23
LC record available at https://lccn.loc.gov/2018009644

Printed in the United States of America.

Contents

Contributors: Contributors: Champions Question and Answer Exhibits   vii
Contributors: Evidence-Based Review Abstracts and Case Examples   ix
Preface   xi
Acknowledgments   xv

SECTION I: CONCEPTS FOR TEACHING AND LEARNING ACROSS DIVERSE TECHNOLOGIES

1   Teaching and Learning With Technologies for Safe, Quality Care   3

2   Keeping Up With Changing Technology, Quality Improvement, and Lifelong Learning   15

3   Models and Theories for Teaching and Learning With Technologies: Systems, Populations, Quality, and Safety Focus   29

4   Technology Teaching and Learning: Engaging Assignments and Lesson Plans   43

5   Evidence-Based Practice: Gaining and Using the Evidence With Technology   57

SECTION II: FACULTY AS LEARNING FACILITATORS WITH TECHNOLOGY

6   Creating Learning Teams: Basics for Safe/Effective Communication   73

7   Technology, Social Spaces, and Teaching and Learning Strategies to Build the Learning Community   89

8   Applied Technologies Assignments: Engaging the Learner for Quality and
Safety   103

9   Engaging the Learner With Technologies for Feedback, Debriefing, and
Evaluation   117

SECTION III: DIVERSE CLINICAL PRACTICE AND EDUCATIONAL TECHNOLOGIES

10   Online Education: Maximizing the Opportunities for Learning Populations
and Systems Care   133

11   Hybrid Learning: The Changing Classroom and Technology to Promote
Quality Care   151

12   Simulation: Creating Safe Environments for Learning Patient Care   165

13   Informatics: Teaching Clinical Data Management for Populations and
Systems Health   181

14   Technology and Clinical Teaching and Learning: Creating a Culture of
Safety   199

15   Engaging Patients and Families for Safe, Quality Patient Care With
Technology   219

16   Special Contexts for Educational Leadership With Technology   237

17   Into the Future: Nurse Educators, Teaching Technologies,
and Self-Directed Lifelong Learning   255

Appendix A: New Technology Readiness Inventory   267
Appendix B: Integrated Learning Triangle for Teaching With Technologies   269
Index   271

Contributors: Champions Question and Answer Exhibits

Chapter 10   Online Education: Maximizing the Opportunities for Learning Populations and Systems Care

Jan Foecke, PhD, MS, RN, ONC
University of Kansas, Kansas City, Kansas

Chapter 11   Hybrid Learning: The Changing Classroom and Technology to Promote Quality Care

Kathleen Ward, MSN, RN
Fort Hays State University, Hays, Kansas

Chapter 12   Simulation: Creating Safe Environments for Learning Patient Care

Breah Chambers, DNP, APRN, FNP-C
University of Kansas, Kansas City, Kansas

Chapter 13   Informatics: Teaching Clinical Data Management for Populations and System Health

Helene Winstanley, PhD, RN, ANP-C, CCRN-K
University of Kansas, Kansas City, Kansas

Chapter 14   Technology and Clinical Teaching and Learning: Creating a Culture of Safety

Megha Bonnel, MSN, APRN
Stormont Vail Regional Medical Center, Topeka, Kansas

Chapter 15   Engaging Patients and Families for Safe, Quality Patient Care With Technology

Martha Baird, PhD, APRN/CNS-BC, CTN-A
University of Kansas, Kansas City, Kansas

Chapter 15   Engaging Patients and Families for Safe, Quality Patient Care With Technology

Katie Crossland, BSN, RN, TCRN
Trego County-Lemke Memorial Hospital, Wakeeney, Kansas

Chapter 16   Special Contexts for Educational Leadership With Technology

Rhonda D. Klaus, MSN, RN
Hays Medical Center, Hays, Kansas

Chapter 16   Special Contexts for Educational Leadership With Technology

Lisa Larson, PhD, RN
University of Kansas, Kansas City, Kansas

Contributors: Evidence-Based Review Abstracts and Case Examples

Chapter 2   Keeping Up With Changing Technology, Quality Improvement, and Lifelong Learning

Evidence-Based Review Abstract: Online Readiness to Learn
Jamie S. Myers, PhD, RN, AOCNS
University of Kansas Medical Center, Kansas City, Kansas

Chapter 3   Models and Theories for Teaching and Learning With Technologies: Systems, Populations, Quality, and Safety Focus

Evidence-Based Review Abstract: Learning to Learn With Concept Mapping
Patricia Conejo, PhD, RN, WHNP
Professor of Nursing, MidAmerica Nazarene University, Olathe, Kansas

Chapter 4   Technology Teaching and Learning: Engaging Assignments and Lesson Plans

Evidence-Based Review Abstract: Best Practice for Orienting Students to Learning
Suzanne Stricklin, PhD, RN, CNE
Professor, Miami University Nursing, School of Engineering and Applied Science, Oxford, Ohio

Chapter 8   Applied Technologies Assignments: Engaging the Learner for Quality and Safety

Evidence-Based Review Abstract: Storytelling as a Teaching and Learning Concept
Cheryl A. Spittler, PhD, RN, CPSN
Quinn Plastic Surgery Center, Overland Park, Kansas

Chapter 9   Engaging the Learner With Technologies for Feedback, Debriefing, and Evaluation

Evidence-Based Review Abstract: Reflective Journaling
Janet Reagor, PhD, RN
Assistant Professor of Nursing, Avila University School of Nursing, Kansas City, Missouri

Chapter 10   Online Education: Maximizing the Opportunities for Learning Populations and Systems Care

Evidence-Based Review Abstract: Seeking Best Evidence and Promoting Online Integrity
Amanda L. Alonzo, PhD, RN
Instructor, Pittsburg State University, Pittsburg, Kansas

Chapter 11   Hybrid Learning: The Changing Classroom and Technology to Promote Quality Care

Evidence-Based Review Abstract: Listening for a "Click" in Classrooms
Shelley D. Barenklau, CRNA, DNP
Clinical Assistant Professor, University of Kansas Department of Nurse Anesthesia Education, Kansas City, Kansas

Chapter 12   Simulation: Creating Safe Environments for Learning Patient Care

Evidence-Based Review Abstract: Faculty Orientation to Learning Simulation
Christine L. Hober, PhD, RN-BC, CNE
Professor, Fort Hays State University, Hays, Kansas

Chapter 14   Technology and Clinical Teaching and Learning: Creating a Culture of Safety

Exhibit 14.1 Case Example: Online DNP Preceptor Studio
Diane Ebbert, PhD, APRN
Kansas City, Kansas

Moya Peterson, PhD, APRN, FNP-BC
Clinical Associate Professor, University of Kansas School of Nursing, Kansas City, Kansas

Exhibit 14.2 Case Example: Pocit Videos: Point-of-Care Instant Teacher
Mary N. Meyer, PhD, APRN
Clinical Associate Professor, University of Missouri School of Nursing, Kansas City, Missouri

Sharon Kumm, MN, RN, CNE
Clinical Associate Professor, University of Kansas School of Nursing, Kansas City, Kansas

Preface

This book is written for new and future faculty seeking to gain good practices to guide their teaching roles with technology. It is unique in that it addresses changing student learning needs with technologies within the changing healthcare system. Teaching and learning concepts throughout the text link to important concepts related to quality and safety issues, population and public health needs, and systems approaches to care.

As clinical professionals, our focus is on helping students keep the public healthy. Health information technology has been described as a top priority for improving healthcare, with goals specific to informing clinical care, interconnecting clinicians, personalizing care, and improving population health. Irrespective of whether working with students at a distance, in the learning laboratories, or classrooms and clinical settings, varied health and educational technologies help us prepare our students, update our staff, and keep our patients safe. Strategies for teaching both with technology and about technology are incorporated into this text. The science of learning literature provides an opportunity to bring the teacher and student together in learning.

New generations of students are part of a technology-savvy world and are familiar and comfortable with technology. Faculty have the opportunity to optimize these student strengths, using technology to help students create meaning in complex clinical education. Major organizations, including the National League for Nursing and American Association of Colleges of Nursing (AACN), have called for faculty to prepare students in technologies.

This text provides opportunities to learn with other disciplines, focusing on the must-know principles for teaching and learning with diverse technologies. Although not all emerging technologies can be addressed in a book or classroom, good teaching and learning practices, as presented, can help move the mission forward. New chapters to this second edition include the technology leader's role in mentoring, promoting curriculum change, and partnering with colleagues in diverse contexts. An additional focus includes engaging students in addressing patient and population needs in health promotion and extending care to home settings.

Whatever the teaching setting, a key concept is making a good fit between student learning objectives, assignments, and selected technology tools. This text uses the Integrated Learning Triangle for Teaching With Technologies to frame and guide decision making. The text is designed to help reflective educators self-assess and confirm that they are teaching the right concepts in the right way in a changing healthcare world. As students prepare to work in high-technology settings, faculty have a responsibility to help them prepare.

OVERVIEW OF TEXT ORGANIZATION

This book is conceptualized in three sections. Section I provides an overview of teaching and learning concepts that have relevance across a variety of technologies and introduces the Integrated Learning Triangle for Teaching With Technologies. Chapter 1 reminds readers of the basics of good teaching practices and blends those practices with technology. Today's cutting-edge technologies will be replaced by newer technology, so concepts of self-directed learning and lifelong learning are reviewed in Chapter 2. In Chapter 3, readers are introduced to concepts and theories that guide teaching with technology and capture significant student learning. Lesson plans are considered in Chapter 4 as tools for organizing a plan to make technology an efficient part of our teaching and students' learning outcomes. With the rapid proliferation of readily available text-based, audio, and video resources, Chapter 5 considers student technology skills and information literacy, now critical competencies in all nursing programs.

Section II assists readers in enhancing their skills as learning facilitators with technology. Chapter 6 considers good communication practices to guide teaching with technologies and facilitate civil, respectful communication in a variety of situations, including clinical implications for safe quality patient care. Chapter 7, acknowledging that learning communities consist of groups of people engaged in common learning goals, provides facilitator strategies, faculty tools, and strategies to help diverse students learn with technologies. Chapter 8 considers the authentic, active learning that is an important part of learning with technology, engaging students via online opportunities and applied assignments. The faculty role in providing student feedback and debriefing is considered as a component of formative evaluation in Chapter 9.

Section III guides faculty in considering that principles of good teaching and learning serve across technologies. Chapter 10 addresses online education with its many unique teaching and learning opportunities. The changing classroom and technology, with emphasis on the blended classroom, is discussed in Chapter 11. Chapter 12, addressing simulated clinical learning experiences, focuses on teaching and learning strategies to help students practice critical thinking and safety competencies in the safety of the clinical laboratory and before students enter fast-paced healthcare settings. Chapter 13 focuses on helping students gain skills with nursing informatics, including the tools of electronic health records (EHRs) to promote patient safety and care quality. Chapter 14 is about teaching clinical technologies, focusing on faculty tools to guide students in the safe, efficient use of clinical technologies and accompanying caring behaviors. Engaging patients and addressing population needs for health promotion are the focus of new Chapter 15. The technology leaders' role in mentoring faculty, promoting needed curriculum change, and partnering with colleagues for technologies sharing is emphasized in Chapter 16. The final chapter, Chapter 17, emphasizes opportunities for using technology projects to further scholarship, engaging interprofessional teams, and reflecting about teaching with technologies into the future. Applications specific to online, classroom, and clinical teaching technologies are shared throughout the text. These topics have relevance for both student and staff development and even patient education. The Institute of Medicine (2003) Health Professions Educator Competencies adapted by Quality and Safety Education for Nurses (QSEN) Institute are integrated in chapter discussions, as well as technology recommendations from AACN, National League for Nursing, and other national groups.

FORMAT AND FEATURES

This book is designed for graduate students, faculty, and staff educators learning to use technologies effectively and efficiently in their teaching. On the basis of science of learning principles, educational theory, and best practices, the text integrates resources from a variety of disciplines. Guided by a chapter goal, each chapter is organized in a time-efficient format with brief text, bullets, and resource exhibits. Faculty come from varied educational settings, with unique resources and diverse student levels, so concepts in this text are presented broadly for faculty to adapt to their own teaching and learning milieus. The following features are included:

Reflective Questions: Each chapter begins and ends with reflective questions to support faculty roles as reflective educators seeking to improve teaching. Introductory reflections are designed to acknowledge and build on readers' past experiences. Ending reflections are designed for self-reflection on new ideas gained from reading and plans for using these ideas.

Integrated Learning Triangle for Teaching With Technologies: A major feature of the text is the Integrated Learning Triangle for Teaching With Technologies. Designed to provide a central organizing tool for lesson planning and decision making, the Integrated Learning Triangle serves as a faculty guide for determining if and how technology can promote student learning. Accompanying questions help address planning needs. Irrespective of whether technology decisions are for an entire course or one assignment, the Integrated Learning Triangle applies across a wide variety of educational and practice technologies from low to high technology.

Chapter Resources and Case Examples: Each chapter provides a variety of Internet resources emphasizing national resources that students can access to stay up to date. Selected chapters include self-assessment tools, case examples, and further resources to promote learning to teach with and about technologies.

Quick Tips: Each chapter ends with quick teaching tips to serve as reminders of important concepts for planning and implementing our teaching and learning activities.

Evidence-Based Review Abstracts: Our focus is teaching and learning with the best evidence, so many chapters provide an evidence summary of a pedagogical concept from synthesized references to highlight best educational practices. For example, topics such as student readiness to learn and promoting online integrity are included.

Champions Question and Answer Exhibits: In an effort to "keep it real," a number of chapters include questions answered by our practice experts or "champions" to address the day-to-day practices they have used in integrating technology into the curriculum.

Online Resources for Further Learning: This text supports lifelong learning, so each chapter includes websites for gaining additional teaching and learning ideas. Although Internet addresses for important resources are supplied in each chapter, URLs may change, so readers are reminded to perform a search by site name or reference to identify a changed address.

In this text, the broad term *technology* encompasses diverse technologies in clinical and classroom settings, in addition to web-based learning tools. In addition, the authors use the word *faculty* interchangeably with personal pronouns because authors continue along with our readers in the teaching with technologies journey.

Nurses have unique roles in using technology both in learning and in caring for patients. The rapid increase in online learning, the call for all students to gain informatics competencies, and the rapid increase in high-fidelity patient simulator use are all examples of the need for faculty to update their skills in technology. This book is designed to help readers appreciate the rapidly changing future of technology and clinical practice, refocusing on the need to be self-directed, lifelong learners. As the authors' own children, truly technology-savvy learners, advance in their educational careers, the authors are often reminded of the important roles that faculty play in helping students to be successful. We hope our readers gain ideas for using technology in promoting the success of many future students!

Wanda E. Bonnel
Katharine Vogel Smith
Christine L. Hober

Acknowledgments

The authors acknowledge all those individuals who have influenced the writing of this book. We especially thank our families for their patience as we pursued writing this book; individuals who have contributed and shared resources for various chapters; our university colleagues for introducing us to many technology resources; and our Springer colleagues, for their encouragement in text development.

Concepts for Teaching and Learning Across Diverse Technologies

Teaching and Learning With Technologies for Safe, Quality Care

CHAPTER GOAL

Gain an overview of teaching with technologies, including an introduction to the text and tools that are used throughout the book to promote teaching and learning with technology.

BEGINNING REFLECTION

1. What experiences have you had teaching and learning with technology?
2. What experiences have you had using technologies for safe, quality patient care?
3. What are your goals for expanding the use of technology in promoting student learning?

Overheard: *Although I am told that teaching with technologies is intuitive, I am not sure I agree....*

Traditional teaching methods have not always kept up with rapidly changing technology. Rapid expansion in online learning, national calls for all students to gain informatics competencies, and the major impact of high-fidelity patient simulators all support the need for faculty competence and confidence in teaching with technologies. Because all levels of faculty seek to enhance traditional teaching with technologies, how do nursing faculty keep up with the rapid changes? This book provides an overview of teaching and learning concepts or pedagogies that are relevant across a variety of technologies. This book can help new and seasoned educators gain strategies for keeping up with technologies. It can also help faculty make thoughtful selections of how and where technology should be integrated into learning environments to meet specific educational goals. Readers can gain new ideas for integrating technology-based learning strategies in their own teaching projects.

Technology and the changing clinical arena are an interesting mix. Addressing technology is important in this time of rapid change in healthcare and renewed emphasis on safety and quality in clinical care. As national reports document problems with communication and safety in the health professions, technology can provide unique opportunities for making improvements in these critical areas. What considerations are necessary in technology integration into healthcare programs? How does technology affect teaching and learning? Basic approaches that are covered in this text include the following:

- Helping our students (and ourselves) recognize personal learning styles and skills for self-directed learning
- Gaining a conceptual tool kit that can promote success in teaching and learning concepts (such as evidence-based practice) with a technology base
- Gaining familiarity with a variety of available teaching resources such as the Quality and Safety Education for Nurses (QSEN) Institute (www.qsen.org)
- Gaining a template for teaching technologies that is based on best-practice evidence

This book is about combining the best of the traditional teaching and learning principles with new, rapidly changing technologies. We have explored the advantages and limits of teaching with and about technologies. We are not expecting our readers to become experts in all technologies. Rather, the idea of the book is to understand good basic teaching and learning principles, educational leadership, and quality and safety practices and to apply them to rapidly changing technologies. This book is intended not to develop skill proficiency with a particular software or technology, but rather to introduce pedagogical concepts and practices relevant to future teaching with technology.

Methods supplied throughout this text are consistent with adult learning theory. In rapidly changing arenas such as educational technology and clinical knowledge, there are benefits to time-tested theory in guiding rapid decision making to meet student and patient needs. This is particularly important for students in clinical professions.

WHY ARE PEDAGOGIES IMPORTANT AND WHAT DO THEY MEAN?

A world of technology has opened up for our use in teaching and learning. In particular, our overall focus on pedagogies has been enhanced by the major shift that online learning presented. As learning moved online, educators were pushed to think of what they were trying to accomplish with teaching rather than just moving a classroom session to the web. As new technologies emerged for both classroom and clinical units, more opportunities to consider pedagogy and technology combinations exist. Although the term andragogy was defined as referring specifically to adult learners (Knowles, 1984), the more common umbrella term pedagogy is used throughout this text. A pedagogical approach reminds us to keep student learning at the forefront. Although varied definitions for pedagogy exist, the term relates to the activities of educating or instructing that facilitate learning by another. The concept of facilitator is the key throughout our discussions.

In addition, best-practice pedagogies relate to learning by doing. Although definitions of best practice can vary, examples of teaching principles and resources based on evidence include the following:

- Chickering and Gamson (1987). This classic reference describes seven best practices for teaching.
- Carnegie Mellon University (2015). In these resources, research-based principles are expanded to include both teaching and learning principles.
- National Academy of Sciences (2015). This resource provides a basic reference on how people learn.

Technology enhances teaching opportunities and, in some cases, may even make teaching easier. Technology, for example, allows ready access to new materials. Gaining knowledge of simulation practices is at our fingertips using the Simulation Innovation Resource Center (SIRC). The question then becomes how to help students know where to look to gain these best tools not only now, but also in future practice.

Approaches to teaching with technologies are quite varied. The meaning of even a seemingly straightforward term such as online course can vary greatly. Our intent is to build opportunities and enhance readers' repertoire of tools for conveying content and using technology when it presents the best solution for helping our students learn. As faculty, we want to not only convey content to our students, but also help them understand what to do with the content so that they can make the connections between concepts and put concepts into context. Determining the best practices to do this is a worthy goal.

WHAT DO WE MEAN BY TECHNOLOGIES?

Technology is a very broad term, and its use in education has been described in different ways. Skiba, Connors, and Jeffries (2008) have considered the term to consist of three frames, including educational technology, information management, and clinical practice technology. Although there is overlap in the three frames, they provide direction for our discussions. We have addressed our teaching from the educational technology frame and consider how best to teach concepts within the practice frames, with an overarching information literacy theme.

Although we are privileged to live in a technology-rich time with all the accompanying opportunities, this fast and furious pace may lead us to question how we can make teaching with technologies manageable. Technology changes too fast to constantly focus and learn updates, so we must focus on the broad concepts or pedagogies that facilitate our use of technologies to promote student learning.

Educational Technologies

Technology provides educational options. We are talking not only about teaching online, but also about the many ways that classroom and clinical activities can be enhanced by technology. For example, we can give students the option of reading texts in print versions or using online teaching resources such as Center for Excellence in the Care of Vulnerable Populations (Brewington, n.d.). Also, assignments traditionally shared in the classroom, such as creating posters or brochures for health fairs, can be developed electronically in teams, viewed electronically, and then debriefed in class or by online discussion. Students can view these documents before class and come ready to debrief in class or in an online discussion. Using this electronic medium not only works for students, but also helps prepare them for using these resources as tools in their clinical practice. We have discussed our resources, courses, and assignments differently. We have used theories and best practices to guide us when research does not keep up with our rapidly changing needs.

Even in our core or basic classes, there are many opportunities for using technology to enhance teaching and learning. In a pathophysiology class, for example, faculty might use technologies to capture self-assessments, present automated quizzes with instant feedback for student learning, apply case studies to make the learning more relevant, engage students with questions embedded in PowerPoint presentations, and assign a relevant clinical project such as teaching handouts or posters to be completed with technology. Follow-up discussions on online discussion boards might be assigned. Ultimately, good teaching principles should align with technology applications for quality student learning. (See Exhibit 1.1.)

Information Management and Clinical Practice Technology

We are taking on expanded roles as we move into teaching technologies in the clinical setting. Technology has populated our clinical worlds in terms of managing information and working with our patients. The Institute for Healthcare Improvement (2017) discusses the triple aim, including

---

EXHIBIT 1.1

HOW MANY WAYS ARE THERE TO TEACH RESPIRATORY ASSESSMENT?

Should all classes on respiratory assessment be taught the same way? Is technology needed to teach assessment? Could technology enhance learning? How many ways can you identify to do each of the following? How do you know what the best approach is?

- How many ways are there to teach respiratory assessment?
- How many ways are there to document a respiratory assessment?
- How many ways are there to encourage critical thinking with a respiratory assessment?
- How might technology (and which technology?) assist with any of these tasks?

improving patient experiences of care, improving health of populations, and reducing the cost of healthcare. Patients are seeking healthcare that is evidence based, meaningful, and personally delivered in settings where technology is used. Technology, such as using electronic medical records to store, manage, retrieve, and analyze data, is key to improving the health of populations. Healthcare professionals gain unique information about populations via electronic data sets. In addition, technology provides opportunity to promote clinical safety, support population health, gain efficiency in teaching and learning, and it makes it easier for health professionals to track information, to get reminders on care issues, and to develop plans for positive patient outcomes. Technology is a tool for facilitating connections, caring, and collaboration.

Four broad technology goals for practice conveyed by the U.S. Department of Health & Human Services (Brailer, 2004) are specific to informing clinical care, interconnecting clinicians, personalizing care, and improving population health. Practice technology not only includes teaching students to care for patients on respirators in the ICU, but also involves changes from paper to electronic patient charting or documentation. In addition, the Institute of Medicine (IOM, 1999) safety report reminds us to use technology for a variety of reasons, including enhanced team communication to promote patient safety and outcomes. Patient safety in common practices such as medication administration and fall prevention is now often promoted with technologies that help assess, monitor, and direct care planning using interprofessional educational practices. Faculty gain opportunity to help students use technology in supporting patient care. Gaining familiarity with diverse technologies for teaching and learning to promote safe student practices and positive patient outcomes is a focus of this text.

The overarching information-literacy theme has particular relevance to our students of the future, serving as a basic platform for all of their professional work. Information literacy serves as guide to faculty for teaching evidence-based practice. As faculty, we first consider where to find best evidence to share with our students and then we teach them how to find their own best evidence for their future practice.

OUR DIVERSE LEARNERS AND THEIR CLINICAL PRACTICE

We have worked with diverse students in the classroom and in clinical units, including students who are diverse both in their cultural backgrounds and in their learning styles and interests. Our students bring a range of academic proficiencies, as well as unique talents and desires, to becoming clinical professionals. As faculty, we are challenged to help all of our students gain learning tools for success. An outcomes orientation in nursing education also includes a focus on the student remediation that technology makes much easier for us to provide.

We are preparing to teach students who will be practicing across diverse settings, from acute care to homes to long-term care. Students provide care ranging from health promotion to palliative care. The amount of information they will need can seem overwhelming unless we use broad concepts to help them learn the must-know content.

THINKING CONCEPTUALLY

Our discussions in this text often relate to the broad concepts that can keep us moving forward with diverse patient populations, rapidly changing clinical settings, and technologies. We are preparing to teach students who will be practicing across diverse settings from acute care to extended care settings and caring for patients from infants to frail elders. Thinking conceptually helps us keep track of broad content areas. Concepts remind us quickly of what we already know about a topic area and lay a foundation for further learning and organizing.

The concepts and themes addressed in this text include teaching about being professional and ethical, using evidence, thinking critically, and being competent in clinical skills. The rapidly changing field of genetics and genomes is one example. Students need to understand the basic concepts of genetics and technology for testing and treatment purposes. Beyond their basic clinical skills, counseling and supporting are called into play. Much of their work in this area relate to having good ethical models for decision making and patient-support strategies, along with an awareness of psychosocial issues and professional practice models.

BUILDING OUR TOOL KIT WITH MODELS AND RESOURCES TO GUIDE TEACHING AND LEARNING

Technology, if used in the best ways, presents opportunities to facilitate many aspects of teaching and learning. Theories and best evidence are our guiding practices in our pedagogies. Adult education reminds us to build on what students already know, engage students in learning the content, apply active relevant assignments, and help motivate students with assignments that incorporate their current and future interests. We learn (and help our students learn) by accessing new information, actively using that information, and reflecting on our learning (Fink, 2013). In addition, specific technology models have helped us synthesize and build on our own skills as faculty as we continue to ask questions and incorporate technologies into our teaching.

Exhibits 1.2 and 1.3 provide two guides for advancing our work with technologies: (a) our Readiness Guide and (b) our Integrated Learning Triangle for Teaching With Technologies. The Readiness Guide provides a checklist approach based on a broad mentoring model (Zachary, 2000) to determine our readiness, opportunities, and motivations for learning about teaching with a particular technology, as well as the opportunities and resources available to us (see Exhibit 1.2). Learning a technology such as Camtasia might be guided

---

EXHIBIT 1.2

NEW TECHNOLOGY READINESS INVENTORY

The following inventory can help answer the why, how, and when of learning a new technology. Organized around the concepts of readiness, opportunity, and support, the inventory provides direction in identifying an individualized plan. Please reflect on the following items specific to a new technology with which you would like to teach.

1. For the *specific* technology, what is your:
   a. Readiness/motivation—What is your readiness to learn/gain comfort with the technology? Would you rate this as low, moderate, or high?
   b. Opportunity—What is available to you in terms of technology resources and environment? Are there opportunities to access the technology you hope to use?
   c. Support—Who is available (locally or at a distance) to mentor or coach you in teaching with a specific technology?
2. Based on your assessment, what learning goals will you set?
   a. Goal statement (includes your intention and time frame).
3. Based on your goals, what specific plan will you design to enhance your technology learning/comfort needs?
   a. Plan (includes two to three specific action steps).
4. What potential challenges exist or might limit your efforts? What strategies would be most likely to promote success?

---

by this checklist of considerations (see Exhibit 1.4). The checklist helps faculty document opportunities and challenges, as well as assess faculty readiness for specific teaching technologies.

As we gain comfort with a particular technology, we may be preparing to design an assignment or a course using it. The Integrated Learning Triangle for Teaching with Technologies, based on best-practice evidence, provides further direction in planning to use technology in teaching. Influenced by the work of Fink (2013), the Integrated Learning Triangle is further clarified around the concepts of BEBOLDER (best evidence, educational theories, beginning assessments, objectives, logistics, decisions, evaluation/feedback, and revisions). This triangle is introduced in Exhibit 1.3 and is referenced in later chapters. The Integrated Learning Triangle helps faculty document opportunities and challenges for student learning, as well as assesses faculty considerations in planning a course, lesson plan, or assignment using technology.

Technology keeps evolving, presenting us with both challenges and opportunities for being flexible and creative. In new areas, where there is limited research, we have to rely on solid theory, educational principles, and best practices. Gaining a tool kit built around broad teaching principles and concepts helps faculty stay flexible and adapt to change. Case examples throughout this text help consider opportunities for using the template with varied content. Promoting the effective and efficient use of a broad array of technologies, the BEBOLDER template sets the stage for lifelong faculty learning and planning that promote student learning with technologies.

EXHIBIT 1.3

INTEGRATED LEARNING TRIANGLE FOR TEACHING WITH TECHNOLOGIES

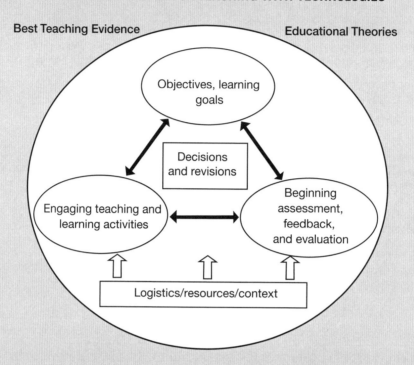

The following guides flow from the Integrated Learning Triangle for Teaching With Technologies and can help answer the why, how, and when of using technology for a specific course, lesson, or assignment. Questions are organized around the mnemonic BEBOLDER to guide reflection. Consider the following items as you think about your plans for using technology:

- *Best* teaching evidence and practices. What evidence is available to guide implementing a particular technology? What are recommended approaches?
- *Educational principles and theories.* What broad principles or theories, such as adult education theory, best fit student learning needs and teaching opportunities?
- *Beginning assessments.* What student learning needs are specific to the student level and content to be taught?
- *Objectives.* What is to be achieved in a specific course, lesson, or assignment? How can technology help?
- *Logistics/context.* What is the setting for teaching and learning? What physical resources are available? How many students are to be engaged? What are the strengths of available resource people to assist them?
- *Decision/fit.* What is the best technology fit for given learning needs and resources? What are the best teaching/learning activities to engage students?
- *Evaluation and feedback.* What is the evaluation plan? What feedback mechanisms are integrated into the course? How will you know if technology is helping students learn?
- *Review and revision.* How will you build quality improvement into your plan? What worked and what did not? What needs to be improved?

(continued)

FURTHER QUESTIONS TO GUIDE REFLECTIONS

How does a particular technology best meet learning needs? For a particular course or assignment, will the technology:

- Help capture the concepts you are teaching?
- Assist students in meeting the objectives of the course?
- Help focus students' learning? Motivate students to become involved in learning?
- Help students make transitions to practice or focus on important concepts?

Also, for a given point in time:

- Is a particular technology worth the time and effort? (Would a less expensive technology work as well? What are the trade-offs?)
- What is the evidence for using the technology? (If there is limited evidence, is it consistent with good theory and educational principles?)
- Is the workload reasonable and well placed for both faculty and students?

EXHIBIT 1.4

LEARNING A TECHNOLOGY: FIRSTHAND ACCOUNT FROM AN ANONYMOUS AUTHOR

As a faculty member seeking to enhance my audio presence with online students, I was seeking opportunities for obtaining a technology and the know-how to use it. Using the Readiness-Opportunity-Support Checklist (see Exhibit 1.2), I gained some ideas for following up on this need. At our university, I found both resources and opportunity for an initial training session to prepare me to learn the new (to me) Camtasia; I was motivated and ready to learn.

After making a special trip to our college, I arrived early and ready to go. (I am now aware there are also online videos of this technology to support my work.) As the session began, I started stressing out because I did not realize the variety of things I could do with the Camtasia technology and thought I had come to the wrong session. Then I calmed down and focused on the parts I wanted. The session helped me confirm that my goal of providing brief audio clips to an online class made sense. I then scheduled a follow-up session with the Camtasia presenter, who had offered further mentoring services. At this follow-up session, I got a sense that my planned project was feasible from a technical standpoint. Then I needed to think about how it was feasible from a pedagogical standpoint. Here is where I started using the Integrated Learning Triangle for Teaching with Technologies to guide me (see Exhibit 1.3).

As I learned Camtasia, I was not starting from scratch. I used teaching skills I have learned throughout my career and have organized around adult education principles. I have created class outlines, and I know how to interact with a group of students to engage them in learning. Key points for me to consider beyond the physical "how-to" of Camtasia now related much more to pulling educational concepts together. Pushing the big red start button on the technology is the least of my worries. Instead, I am focusing on organizing manageable content bites that will encourage students in their own readings and activities. I am thinking about tricky concepts that I could describe in additional content bites. I am considering how to make the information relevant to the students with my examples and theirs.

SUMMARY

This is a book about understanding teaching technologies in partnership with pedagogy. We are being asked to teach in new ways that differ from the ways in which we were taught. New approaches are also needed for educating ourselves in using technology. Technology will continue to be a moving target, so we need to focus on pedagogy and student learning goals, building the technology around goals to support learning. As technology changes, we can tweak our technology skills and continue to use our educational principles and best practices. As educators reflecting on our practice, we consider questions for ongoing thought and learning resources with each chapter. Our goal is to share guides for keeping up with teaching technologies without being overwhelmed. Ideas and activities for self-directed learning are incorporated throughout the text.

ENDING REFLECTIONS FOR YOUR LEARNING NOTEBOOK

1. What is the most important content that you learned in this chapter?
2. What are your plans for using the information provided in this chapter in your future teaching endeavors?
3. What are your further learning goals?

GUIDELINES FOR TEACHING AND LEARNING WITH TECHNOLOGIES

Quick Teaching Tips

1. Orient students to their learning responsibilities and self-directed learning opportunities at the beginning of class.
2. Gain familiarity with web-based resources designed to support faculty in teaching with technologies such as QSEN Institute resources (available online at http://qsen.org/faculty-resources/courses/learning-modules).

Questions for Further Reflection

1. Using Exhibit 1.2 as a resource, think about what specific new technology you would like to learn about given your readiness/motivation, opportunity, and support services to enhance your technology learning/comfort needs.
2. Think back on how you were taught respiratory assessment. How would you recommend teaching the content with technology for diverse students?

Learning Activity: Self-Reflection on Technologies

As you begin your work in teaching with technologies, consider the following self-assessment, indicating Agree or Disagree for each of the following statements. As you review further chapters (or discuss the survey with colleagues), see if your opinions change or stay the same.

1. ____Helping students become self-directed learners takes on increasing importance in teaching with technologies.
2. ____Active learning has limited relevance for online courses/classes.
3. ____Technology has made information literacy and searching the literature easier concepts for students to understand.
4. ____Technology is advanced using interprofessional collaboration.
5. ____Electronic medical records can serve as tools to promote student critical thinking.
6. ____Student–faculty boundary setting has gotten easier with online social spaces such as Facebook and Snapchat.
7. ____Students in observer roles, as well as students with actual case roles, can learn with simulation.
8. ____Clickers in the classroom promote opportunities for gaining test-taking skills.
9. ____Fall-safety projects have little to do with teaching data management.
10. ____Rubrics, in addition to evaluation, serve as effective student learning tools.
11. ____Technology provides numerous ways to organize and facilitate student clinical work.
12. ____Students need opportunities to learn critique of web-based audiovisuals.

Learning Activity: Create an Assignment

BEBOLDER—CONCEPT MAP

The purpose of this assignment is to practice using the Integrated Learning Triangle for Teaching With Technologies with a teaching topic of interest.

After studying the Integrated Learning Triangle for Teaching With Technologies (Exhibit 1.3) model, develop a concept map depicting a topic (e.g., assessing lung sounds) that you would like to teach for a course, lesson, or assignment. Consider your responses to the questions framed by BEBOLDER. Once you have responded to the questions related to your teaching topic, depict them on a concept map. What strengths and weaknesses do you see with your plan?

Online Resources for Further Learning

- Technology Informatics Guiding Education Reform (TIGER) Initiative (Health Information Technology). This site describes the TIGER competencies and suggested targets for knowledge, skill, and attitude development during prelicensure education. www.tigersummit.com

- QSEN Institute. A Robert Wood Johnson Foundation Initiative, this project provides interesting tools and resources to promote student learning, located at www.qsen.org
- NLN Center for Excellence in the Care of Vulnerable Populations. This site currently discusses the unique needs of adults, veterans, and Alzheimer's patients with the caregivers in the initiative Advancing Care Excellence (ACE). www.nln.org/centers-for-nursing-education/nln-center -for-excellence-in-the-care-of-vulnerable-populations
- SIRC. This site offers courses on designing and debriefing in simulations, interprofessional education (IPE), and advanced evaluation. sirc.nln.org

REFERENCES

Brewington, J. (n.d.). NLN Center for Excellence in the Care of Vulnerable Populations. Retrieved from http://www.nln.org/centers-for-nursing-education/nln-center-for-excellence-in-the-care-of-vulnerable -populations2

Carnegie Mellon University. (2015). Theory and research-based principles of learning. Retrieved from https://www.cmu.edu/teaching/principles/learning.html

Chickering, A. W., & Gamson, Z. F. (1987). Seven principles for good practice in undergraduate education. Retrieved from https://files.eric.ed.gov/fulltext/ED282491.pdf

Fink, L. D. (2013). *Creating significant learning experiences: An integrated approach to designing college courses* (2nd ed.). San Francisco, CA: Jossey-Bass.

Institute of Medicine (1999). *To err is human: Building a safer health system*. Washington, DC: National Academies Press.

Institute for Healthcare Improvement. (2017). IHI triple aim initiative. Retrieved from http://www.ihi .org/Engage/Initiatives/TripleAim/Pages/default.aspx

Knowles, M. S. (1984). *Andragogy in action: Applying modern principles of adult education*. San Francisco, CA: Jossey-Bass.

National Academy of Sciences. (2015). *Reaching students: What research says about effective instruction in undergraduate science and engineering*. Washington, DC: National Academies Press.

Skiba, D. J., Connors, H. R., & Jeffries, P. R. (2008). Information technologies and the transformation of nursing education. *Nursing Outlook, 56*(5), 225–230. doi:10.1016/j.outlook.2008.06.012

U.S. Department of Health and Human Services. (2004). The decade of health information technology: Delivering consumer-centric and information-rich health care. Retrieved from https://permanent .access.gpo.gov/gpo800/hitframework.pdf

Zachary, L. J. (2000). *The mentor's guide: Facilitating effective learning relationships*. San Francisco, CA: Jossey-Bass.

CHAPTER 2

Keeping Up With Changing Technology, Quality Improvement, and Lifelong Learning

CHAPTER GOAL

Gain practical tips for using self-directed learning, quality improvement, and technologies for lifelong learning.

BEGINNING REFLECTION

1. What experiences have you had with self-directed learning?
2. How do you practice, teach, and encourage others to be lifelong learners?
3. How might technologies assist in quality improvement?

Overheard: *I would like to update the technologies I use in my courses, but where should I start?*

Clinical knowledge is changing rapidly with the advent of technology. Faculty can no longer hope to convey all clinical information to students in the classroom. At best, faculty can assist students in learning broad concepts and then prepare them to keep up with the changing details. The concepts of self-directed learning (SDL) and lifelong learning are critical in our technology-rich age. SDL is a tool that the clinical professionals need today. Knowledge gained by the students in our courses rapidly become out of date if we do not help them acquire skills as self-directed, lifelong learners. This chapter discusses SDL, especially as it relates to teaching with technologies.

Technology provides opportunities for dealing with the complex and massive information presented to us daily. Quality improvement is an example of continued information management that uses technology for the intent of improving a situation or process. Technologies play a key role in keeping up and managing our ongoing learning and improvement needs. For both faculty and students, the web is an essential tool for lifelong learning. Acknowledging that faculty will have students for just a short time in classes, it is imperative that we teach them skills to maintain a knowledge base as clinicians. In this chapter, strategies for engaging ourselves and our students as lifelong learners are described.

WHAT DO WE MEAN BY SDL?

Knowles (1975) identified a self-directed learner as an adult who seeks to take learning initiative, diagnose learning needs, formulate learning goals, identify learning resources, and choose or implement learning plans and evaluation. SDL as a component of adult education has been documented extensively by Hiemstra and Brockett (1994) in early work. A related concept, lifelong learning has been described as a process of learning that depends on individual needs, as well as interests and learning skills, and that continues throughout a lifetime (Hiemstra, 2002). For our discussion, lifelong learning is considered a continuation or part of SDL.

Understanding what SDL means to different individuals provides the beginning of teaching and learning direction. SDL is not, as the term might suggest, focused on totally independent study and learning. The concept of SDL can be considered from a variety of perspectives and may mean different things to different people. For many classes, SDL is only one aspect of the course. For example:

- In clinical laboratories, SDL might mean asking students to prepare independently for a check-off as part of varied clinical assignments.
- In the classroom setting, SDL may mean choosing a project to complete from a menu of options.
- At a distance education site, SDL might mean completing self-directed modules via the web.

The SDL concept has taken on increased relevance with the advent of online learning and the need to coach students at a distance in their learning activities. Assigning beginning students a large textbook and telling them to "know everything" is obviously not the intent of SDL. It is important to know that SDL is not an all-or-nothing concept, SDL does not imply learning in isolation, and SDL is not an easy way for faculty to opt out of teaching (Hiemstra & Brockett, 1994).

Are SDL and lifelong learning the same thing? The two concepts seem to be quite similar. The authors, for example, have used technology as a part of SDL since graduate school, when first going to the library to find the required references and then to the copy machine to create copies for further reading. Although SDL approaches have changed over the years, the authors believe that they gained the basics of identifying a need, a plan, and tools as SDL and have since used these skills as lifelong learners. It seems that SDL and lifelong learning are similar concepts with a "time" focus built in.

SDL can vary from simple learning choices to the creation of full independent study courses. For our purposes as educators, the SDL discussion is twofold. First, SDL helps learners see their role in learning while they become more accountable for their own learning. Second, SDL involves helping learners enhance their enthusiasm, skill set, and resources for becoming lifelong learners. This second discussion provides student learning tools or competencies required by all students, such as information literacy. Without this competency, students are not able to keep using evidence-based practice in their future clinical roles.

SDL includes being proactive in gaining skills for ongoing learning. Fink (2013) discussed the importance of identifying oneself as a learner and the importance of learning how to learn. Motivating ourselves and our students to be lifelong learners is the key. Selected aspects of SDL include the following (Hiemstra & Brockett, 1994):

- SDL includes a sense of appreciating learning skills and valuing learning opportunities.
- There are different degrees of SDL, ranging from simple assignment choices to creating objectives and plans for an independent study.
- SDL involves helping students learn to self-assess and identify what they know and what they still need to know (i.e., knowledge gaps) about a specific concept.
- SDL incorporates helping students gain tools, techniques, and resources that support learning and accessing this information for knowledge gaps.
- SDL involves a student–faculty partnership approach to learning and differs from a traditional classroom lecture approach in which students may be somewhat passive learners.

As noted, SDL can be considered broadly and varies from students who are provided some direction and opportunities for assignment choice and those who take primary responsibility for their learning plans. The goal for most courses is to help students take a more active role and accountability for their learning so that graduates accept responsibility for their own SDL. Once students comprehend the implications and inherent value of SDL, the skill set of being an SDL can evolve into processes for lifelong learning. Nursing, like other practice disciplines, requires lifelong learning to keep abreast of technological advances and the provision of high-quality, safe healthcare services.

THEORY BACKGROUND FOR SDL

Adult education and SDL are closely related. Adult education concepts include building on the past experiences of the learner, making content relevant, and making content applicable and useful for the learner. Consistent with SDL, as students learn about a new respiratory illness, for example, they are reminded to build on past coursework and experiences with basic structural and functional concepts of the respiratory system learned in core science courses. Building from the foundational concepts, faculty guide students in considering the best resource for gaining the relevant content, and then in applying the new information with cases and quizzes that will be relevant to practice.

SDL is not a linear approach to learning; rather, it is complex. SDL concepts are consistent with constructivist learning theory, which supports the fact that students "construct" learning or the knowledge gained to fit their contexts. The individual uses the information and becomes the owner of knowledge. Students are ultimately in control of accepting and incorporating information into their own experiences. For faculty then, a better comprehension of students' past experiences with and current understanding of specific content is key to supporting student learning. Learner assessments can help identify where the gaps or problems are.

LEARNING ASSESSMENTS, BENCHMARKS, AND PLANS FOR SDL

In its most basic form, SDL is based on self-assessments with benchmarks, learning resources, and a plan that helps achieve learning goals. For faculty as learners, these tools provide a way to consider what we already know, what we still need to know, and what we need to learn (strategies for improving important deficits). We as faculty can begin by focusing on our own learning self-assessment that involves evaluating current knowledge in our content areas based on the accepted benchmarks. Identifying resources and learning plans can then guide us. After gaining this skill set for ourselves, our focus can be how we can best help our students do the same.

Learning Assessments

Learning assessments provide baseline data for creating our learning plans. To complete a learning assessment, we need to know how to self-assess against a standard. As a faculty we identify standards for our clinical and educator competencies. We take stock of our own knowledge deficits, for example, in teaching with technologies. The learning activities presented in this book provide broad approaches to guide faculty reflections related to selected educator topics.

Learning Benchmarks

Benchmarks (consistent with criteria or standards) are basic elements or part of completing learning assessments. In education, for example, entire books, including a classic work by Bailey (1981), have been written about teacher self-assessment against designated benchmarks. Teaching and learning self-assessment standards or competencies for those teaching clinical courses might also come from sources such as the National League for Nursing (NLN). The competencies drafted by this organization serve as a benchmark for guiding classroom teachers in self-assessing (NLN, 2013).

The NLN is a premier organization for faculty and leaders in nursing education. It provides professional development competencies for nurse educators to assess self-practice and teaching practices. Teaching competencies are intended to guide curriculum design and attempt to ensure that all members of the public receive safe, quality care. In addition, Nurse Educator competencies promote excellence in the advanced specialty role of the academic nurse educator by creating criteria for faculty to demonstrate the complexity of the faculty role (NLN, 2013).

Clinical Benchmarks

Clinical benchmarks or competencies are also important to the faculty. Clinical self-assessment may include using "informal" or web-based educational systems. Those seeking standards for addressing clinical competencies such as geriatrics might seek standards provided by national geriatric organizations such as the American Geriatrics Society. Competencies depend on our current role focus and accepted standards of practice at a point in time. National professional organizations and healthcare associations publish competencies, including the Quality and Safety Education for Nurses (QSEN) Institute, Technology Informatics Guiding Education Reform (TIGER) Initiative, and the American Health Information Management Association (AHIMA). See a sample guide for learning assessment in this chapter's Learning Activity.

- The QSEN Institute (2017), funded by the Robert Wood Johnson Foundation, defines prelicense and graduate practice competencies for patient-centered care, teamwork and collaboration, evidence-based practice, quality improvement, safety, and informatics. The overall goal of the QSEN Institute is to better prepare nurses with the knowledge, skills, and attitudes (KSAs) necessary to continuously improve the quality and safety of healthcare systems. The QSEN Institute provides online access to teaching and learning content.
- The TIGER initiative (Healthcare Information and Management Systems Society, 2018) provides competencies for nursing informatics. Nursing should actively advance the national healthcare information technology (IT) agenda using multidisciplinary collaboration, improvement strategies, and commitment to the provision of safer, higher-quality patient care.
- The AHIMA describes a robust set of functions and opportunities for practicing professionals. Because of the widespread and increasing adoption of technology-based information, such as electronic medical records, AHIMA focuses on competencies for data capture, validation, and maintenance to better serve patients, professionals, leaders, and organizations.

Learning Plans

In part, this book helps us, as faculty, be self-directed in designing our own "teaching with technology" plans and learning tasks. This book provides concepts that are important to consider in our teaching. The Readiness-Opportunity-Support (ROS) Checklist (Exhibit 1.2), for example, is available to assess your resources, opportunities, and support for learning a new technology. Readers decide the topics for your projects and activities. The Integrated Learning Triangle for Teaching With Technologies (Exhibit 1.3) serves as a tool for further planning teaching approaches. For example, if you want to learn more for making changes in a physical assessment course (whether online or in the classroom), you can use physical assessment as the background or context for a majority of your thoughts as you read this text.

You are guided to think about how (or if) technologies would help achieve learning goals. You can create a package of experiences that are relevant for your teaching and learning needs. Further detail on using learning contracts as a form of SDL are provided in a detailed 12-step model by Hiemstra (2002).

INTRODUCING QUALITY IMPROVEMENT

Quality improvement is vital in evidence-based healthcare. Quality improvement science is founded in a systematic, standardized, and rigorous process that applies research to healthcare practice and services (Hall & Roussel, 2017). The evolution of quality has transitioned from reactive to proactive, including awareness, improvement strategies, and sustainment to build a culture of safety with continuous quality improvement. Quality improvement is best accomplished in multidisciplinary teams who analyze quality assurance using statistical analysis and systematic frameworks to measure desired and undesired quality and safety outcomes.

Quality improvement requires leaders who are engaged in the process and can serve as driving forces for quality and safety. Collaboration among team members to provide quality patient care as discussed in the IOM (2001) report, *Crossing the Quality Chasm*. Clinical nurses should be able to serve as leaders who develop and implement quality- and safety-improvement projects from inception to completion. Some commonly used quality-improvement models include

- The Donabedian (2003) system model includes structure, process, and outcome concepts. For a healthcare system, the structure, including the healthcare environment, has numerous processes or steps in the provision of care or services. Healthcare outcomes then relate to the combined components of the system's structure and process. Addressing each of the concepts in the system model helps better understand the healthcare systems' comprehensive ability to provide quality care.
- The PDSA model has four key cycles: plan, do, study, and act. PDSA cycles are typically used for rapid cycle of improvement projects.
- The PBED model includes plan, brief, execute, and debrief. Communication skills and team training are part of the various model steps to foster safe care practices.

■ TeamSTEPPS, or Team Strategies and Tools to Enhance Performance and Patient Safety, incorporates human factors, with skill development supporting leadership, collaboration, and communication.

Quality improvement processes are needed in personal self-analysis and in clinical practice. Professional growth in competencies requires systematic review and planned improvement strategies. Quality improvement is inclusive in reflective practice for SDL.

FACULTY ROLE, HELPING STUDENTS BECOME SELF-DIRECTED LEARNERS

Being a Coach

Teaching toward ongoing lifelong learning requires faculty to take on new roles, including coach or facilitator of student learning. Faculty must transition from a more traditional lecturer role to a role that emphasizes building teaching and learning partnerships with students. A coaching role in working with students provides opportunity to help students frame and focus important course concepts. Consistent with the coach analogy, faculty not only support students in their individual learning, but also bring them together as a learning team.

We can help students identify knowledge needs and assist them in identifying learning tasks and selected approaches to gain requisite knowledge. Faculty do more than pass on information; they provide resources and rubrics to guide expected outcomes. Our faculty role with teaching technologies involves helping students understand what they need to know and how to access that information. Faculty provide opportunities for students to gain new information and do something with this information in the form of assignments. Faculty coaches or facilitators help students move forward, assisting and providing the resources they need.

The idea is to encourage and provide student assignments that help students learn about concepts in engaging ways. In a nursing course, for example, the instructor may guide individual learning by providing specific active learning assignments. The instructor may also provide a menu of activities or assignments designed to achieve course outcomes; students can choose the they activities that they find most relevant and meaningful.

In a face-to-face class, faculty might provide assignments that engage students in reviewing a specific healthcare organization such as the online Alzheimer's Association. Students have opportunity to learn to actively review a website and seek evidence-based resources that they can use with current and future patients. Once students are aware of this resource, they have access to the information well after they have left a course. As intended, students will transfer their learning from the classroom to their clinical work.

As noted, a faculty facilitator or coach role in SDL is very different from just handing students books, telling them to learn the information, and then giving and grading a test. Orientation to learning, student reflective self-assessments, and motivational strategies are important concepts in our tool kit and apply to many aspects of teaching and learning.

Orientating Students to SDL

An orientation can provide a framework for student learning in a course. This orientation includes not only learning about or previewing course activities, but also familiarizing students to the various learning tools, assignment plans, and testing plans that will be used. As noted by Fink (2013), students should understand why and how these tools are important in helping them learn their profession.

A good orientation frames the class, providing students with guides about what they will be learning, what the course process will be, what course outcomes are, and what should happen during the course, including how technologies will work. Orientation includes helping students identify the best learning resources available for their role as self-directed learner, including course tools such as textbooks. A one-page class organizer may be provided that synthesizes and gives all directions such as what the course is about and how it will proceed. Orientation frameworks can give students ideas for their own learning plans.

In a study that surveyed students about their perceptions of high-fidelity simulation experiences (Conejo, 2009), for example, students reported wanting orientation information that included the following: What is the main theme of the laboratory? What is expected of us? What skills do we need? Where are things? How do things work? Will we have an actual patient chart? What are the rules? Is this for learning or testing? Providing a good orientation allows students to prepare and understand their role as partners in learning.

Guiding Students via Reflective Self-Assessments

Reflective self-assessments are important tools in SDL, providing students one way to consider what they do and do not know and what they need to further learn. Whether online or in face-to-face classes, Fink (2013) noted that one relatively easy way to both engage students and extend learning includes asking our students to complete self-reflections. Reflection provides the opportunity for students to integrate new information into their own experiences. Reflection, an active process in which students consider their experiences, helps students think about what they are learning. Although this has been noted as particularly relevant in online courses, it has relevance across all types of classes and technologies for better preparing our students.

Reflective exercises add an active component to learning that provides opportunity for students to synthesize and share their experiences with others and further cement learning. Fink (2013) noted that significant learning is enhanced as students reflect on their activities. Reflection can enhance self-evaluation skill as students build on previous experiences and reflect on how an assignment contributed to their learning.

Self-assessments are a form of reflection and are a good place to start an educational endeavor. Self-assessments against a standard help students gain skills in judging the quality of their work; they judge their self-knowledge and determine when more learning is needed.

Self-assessments help determine what has been learned and what still needs to be achieved. However, students need a criterion or standards to self-assess against. The key points are to help students know the most respected standard and reference sources. Rubrics that summarize the key points for learning (either before or after class) provide direction. In addition, portfolios provide a way to record reflections over time.

A variety of technologies from clickers to online surveys provide simple tools with preclass questions that can provide faculty with their students' background information on the topic. Asking students to reflect and share experiences about the concept to be discussed is a type of self-assessment.

Learning style assessments are another aspect of self-assessment because they help students recognize their learning styles and ways to best set up study plans that match their styles. Students can determine if they are visual learners, auditory learners, hands-on learners, or some mix (Fleming, 2009). For example, recognizing they are visual learners and that they can best learn/recall visually displayed information can promote successful student learning plans. Gaining this information can help students identify best strategies and begin learning plans. Exhibit 2.1 provides examples of learning styles inventories that students can complete.

Motivating Students Toward SDL

Students learn more if they care about what they are learning. Svinicki (2005) notes that goal orientation is situation specific. Consistent with adult education and authentic learning, striving to keep learning interesting and relevant

---

EXHIBIT 2.1

LEARNING ASSESSMENTS FOR BEGINNING SDL

Use the following resources to help students gain familiarity with their learning styles:

- How do I learn best? Complete the VARK assessment for a determination of your learning style (http://vark-learn.com/english/page.asp?p=questionnaire).
- How can I build study skills based on my learning style? After completing the VARK assessments, refer to the VARK help sheets specific to your learning styles to gain ideas for your learning plans (http://vark-learn.com/the-vark-questionnaire).

SDL, self-directed learning; VARK, visual aural read/write kinesthetic.

EXHIBIT 2.2

ENCOURAGE A SUCCESSFUL ORIENTATION TO LEARNING

- Develop assignments based on knowledge and skills that are worth learning.
- Create learning tasks for students that just exceed an anticipated base capability but are still within their reach; expect them to succeed.
- Encourage the building of a community of learners in your class, where everyone supports everyone else's attempt to learn.
- Make the classroom a safe place for learning, responding to students' attempts to learn in a caring way.
- If possible, give the learners some choices in what or the way they learn (learning assignments).
- Be a good model of a success-oriented learner in your own scholarship.

Source: Adapted from Svinicki, M. D. (2005). Student goal orientation, motivation, and learning. Retrieved from https://www .ideaedu.org/Portals/0/Uploads/Documents/IDEA%20Papers/IDEA%20Papers/Idea_Paper_41.pdf

---

relate to student motivation. Whether teaching a class, course, or program, it helps to begin by thinking about how to get students to care and be enthused about the topic, as well as ready to join class conversations. A physical therapy assistant (PTA) program provides an example. The summer before the PTA program started, the student received a very upbeat letter introducing him to the program and school. Before school started, he was a student member in the national professional organization and knew what kinds of things he would be doing in the first few weeks of his class. This was a highly motivated young man who headed off to the school.

Providing learning activity choices is consistent with adult education theory, helping make assignments more relevant to students' needs and interests. Providing learning activity choices promotes autonomy and motivation (Hofer, 2013). The importance of building on intrinsic motivation and expectancy of success is also noted by Svinicki (2005). She describes concepts ranging from meaningful learning activities to choice in assignments to promote goal orientation and to create an attitude of learning mastery and expectancy of success (see further examples promoting a success orientation to learning, Exhibit 2.2). Students might, for example, create pamphlets for clinical patients or develop study resources to share with peers on topics that have an immediate relevance for them. Problem-solving assignments serve as motivators in increasing student curiosity. Creative teaching strategies that highlight a variety of authentic activities can motivate active learning in health profession courses (Herrman, 2016).

Building SDL into the "what next" aspect of learning, Fink (2013) describes the importance of helping students set further learning goals. Motivation comes as a function of goals and expectations, so it benefits students to set learning goals and evaluate for progress periodically or at the course end (Hofer, 2013). Encouraging students to take ownership of their learning outcomes or consider who the learning belongs to (Walvoord & Anderson, 2009) helps to avoid an "us/them" dichotomy that can develop with teacher-controlled grades. Helping students consider how they can partner with faculty to enhance their learning is a goal of SDL.

SDL, TECHNOLOGY, AND ENRICHMENT OR REMEDIATION

In addition, technology provides an opportunity for using SDL in student enrichment or remediation. A good example of SDL and technology is students' use of computers for practice testing. Computer-based practice testing provides ongoing learning opportunities rather than just testing. Online testing programs such as ATI (Assessment Technology Institute) Nursing Education and Kaplan provide opportunity for students' SDL. Students, if properly oriented, can get the benefits of knowing where their weaknesses are and what learning areas they need to focus on. This is very different from testing in which students are seeking a grade and are unclear about whether they are performing well. The judicious use of automated practice tests can provide immediate feedback on individual answers and broader individualized learning plans with areas of study outlined.

An evidence-based review abstract, Orientation to Online Learning is shared in Exhibit 2.3. This systematic review provides faculty direction for developing orientation programs using online learning courses and student readiness to learn as exemplar.

EXHIBIT 2.3

EVIDENCE-BASED REVIEW ABSTRACT: ONLINE READINESS TO LEARN

Compiled by Jamie S. Myers, PhD, RN, AOCNS

The following summary provides a graduate student's experience conducting an evidence-based review on the topic of student readiness to learn.

Online education is becoming ever more prevalent across a variety of degree programs and other venues for nursing education, such as staff development and continuing education. Not all nurses are computer savvy and many express frustrations related to lack of expertise. Identification of best practices for online education is important to the nursing community, as is the assessment of nurses' readiness to learn in the online environment. A systematic literature review was performed to explore the teaching and learning concept of online readiness to learn. PubMed, CINAHL, and ERIC databases were searched for the following broad terms: readiness to learn, e-learning readiness, web-based learning readiness, online readiness, orientation for staff development, online learning, and web-based learning. References published in 2000 or later were accepted.

Search results were summarized in an annotated bibliography, with two primary themes emerging: technological readiness and behavioral readiness to learn. Technological readiness involves learners' skill and competence with computers; access to sufficient hardware, software, and Internet access; and administrative support of dedicated time for online education. Behavioral readiness is dependent on a number of concepts such as self-directedness, motivation, self-discipline, and autonomy. These characteristics were reported to be necessary for success with online learning. Strong

(continued)

recommendations were made for both technological and behavioral readiness assessment before initiating online course work. Information gleaned from the systematic literature review was used to design a model case. Using concepts of self-directed learning and adult education principles, a program to promote success in the online learning environment for RNs pursuing a BSN was suggested. Based on the literature, a number of active learning components were included to engage the learner. Participants would be asked to complete the following self-directed activities: download assigned readings from a specific website, use a web link to a program to conduct a self-assessment of their particular learning style (i.e., VARK), complete a self-reflection paper describing personal strengths and opportunities for growth in online learning skills, and participate in the online discussion board to share concrete plans for enhancing the skills necessary for online learning. Grading rubrics are suggested to evaluate achievements. Future research could explore the relation of these strategies to increased online program completion.

SUMMARY

The concepts of SDL and lifelong learning are closely linked and will become increasingly important for students and faculty in our rapidly changing clinical worlds. Technology resources provide opportunities to enhance our faculty roles in both using and teaching SDL for lifelong learning. Teaching tools such as orientations, reflective self-assessments, and assignments that help motivate students provide initial direction. Quality improvement is a process inclusive in reflective practice for lifelong learning. Keeping up with evidence-based resources of the future and continuing to provide quality care to our patients means that SDL is a needed skill.

ENDING REFLECTIONS FOR YOUR LEARNING NOTEBOOK

1. What is the most important content that you learned in this chapter?
2. What are your plans for using the information in this chapter in your future teaching endeavors?
3. What are your further learning goals?

GUIDELINES FOR TEACHING AND LEARNING WITH TECHNOLOGIES

Quick Teaching Tips

1. Provide orientation guides at the beginning of a course. Include orientation to textbooks and technology resources (highlighting key features of each), as well as course content.
2. Have students complete self-assessments on study and learning skills from online resources and set further learning goals.

3. Provide online calendars with assignment dates and encourage students to plot out their study times.
4. When possible, provide students with an opportunity to choose an assignment from a brief lists of options that all meet objectives.

Questions for Further Reflection

1. What level and time is the best to introduce students to concepts of SDL?
2. How would you suggest providing learning activities that are consistent with adult education theory?
3. Which quality-improvement model is most useful in your practice?

Learning Activity: Self-Assessment

The purpose of this activity is to self-assess your current role, capabilities, and comfort with teaching with technologies. Begin this activity by rating yourself on the following questions (Low, Medium, and High)?

1. I can describe the current role of technologies in my teaching._____
2. I have a good "basics" technology tool kit._____
3. I have interest in increasing my technology tool kit._____
4. I can name theories that guide my teaching with technology._____
5. I am comfortable blending my current teaching strategies with new technologies._____
6. I am confident in my skills as a self-directed learner._____

Based on your rating, what initial plan will you generate for your own SDL? How will you use the readiness tool (Exhibit 1.2) and the Integrated Learning Triangle for Teaching With Technologies (Exhibit 1.3) to assist in your planning?

Online Resources for Further Learning

- NLN. This premier organization provides tools and resources for nursing education, including nurse educator competencies. www.nln.org/about/overview
- QSEN Institute. A Robert Wood Johnson Initiative, this project provides interesting tools and resources to promote prelicensure and graduate competencies. www.qsen.org
- The TIGER (Technology Informatics Guiding Education Reform) Initiative (2018). Healthcare Information and Management Systems Society (HIMSS). www.himss.org/professionaldevelopment/tiger-initiative
- AHIMA. AHIMA's Query Toolkit offers the necessary guidelines for successful querying, including templates to guide organizations and professionals in developing their query process. www.ahima.org

REFERENCES

Bailey, G. D. (1981). *Teacher self-assessment: A means for improving classroom instruction.* Washington, DC: National Education Association.

Conejo, P. E. (2009). *Faculty and student perceptions of preparation for and implementation of high fidelity simulation experiences in associate degree nursing programs.* Doctoral Dissertation, University of Kansas.

Donabedian, A. (2003). *An introduction to quality assurance in health care.* New York, NY: Oxford University Press.

Fink, L. D. (2013). *Creating significant learning experiences: An integrated approach to designing college courses* (2nd ed.). San Francisco, CA: Jossey-Bass.

Fleming, N. (2009). The VARK questionnaire. How do I learn best? Retrieved from http://vark-learn.com/the-vark-questionnaire

Hall, H. R., & Roussel, L. A. (2017). *Evidence-based practice: An integrative approach to research, administration, and practice* (2nd ed.). Burlington, MA: Jones & Bartlett.

Healthcare Information and Management Systems Society. (2018). The TIGER initiative. Retrieved from http://www.himss.org/professionaldevelopment/tiger-initiative

Herrman, J. W. (2016). *Creative teaching strategies for the nurse educator* (2nd ed.). Philadelphia, PA: F. A. Davis.

Hiemstra, R. (2002). *Lifelong learning: An exploration of adult and continuing education within a setting of lifelong learning needs* (3rd ed.). Fayetteville, NY: HiTree Press.

Hiemstra, R., & Brockett, R. G. (Eds.). (1994). *Overcoming resistance to self-direction in adult learning.* San Francisco, CA: Jossey-Bass.

Hofer, B. (2013). Motivation in the college classroom. In W. J. McKeachie & M. Svinicki (Eds.), *McKeachie's teaching tips: Strategies, research, and theory for college and university teachers* (14th ed.). Boston, MA: Houghton Mifflin.

Institute of Medicine (2001). *Crossing the quality chasm: A new health system for the 21st century.* Washington, DC: The National Academies Press. doi:10.17226/10027

Knowles, M. S. (1975). *Self-directed learning: A guide for learners and teachers.* New York, NY: Association Press.

National League for Nursing. (2013). Nurse educator core competency. Retrieved from http://www.nln.org/professional-development-programs/competencies-for-nursing-education/nurse-educator-core-competency

Quality and Safety Education for Nurses. (2017). QSEN competencies. Retrieved from http://qsen.org/competencies

Svinicki, M. D. (2005). Student goal orientation, motivation, and learning. Retrieved from https://www.ideaedu.org/Portals/0/Uploads/Documents/IDEA%20Papers/IDEA%20Papers

Walvoord, B. E., & Anderson, V. J. (2009). *Effective grading: A tool for learning and assessment.* San Francisco, CA: Jossey-Bass.

CHAPTER 3

Models and Theories for Teaching and Learning With Technologies: Systems, Populations, Quality, and Safety Focus

CHAPTER GOAL

Recognize the relationship between theories and best practices and their combined impact on both quality teaching with technologies and quality healthcare.

BEGINNING REFLECTION

1. What are your experiences using models and theories?
2. What education-related models and theories do you use?
3. What other models and theories supplement the use of educational theories to inform your teaching and learning with technology?
4. What is your familiarity with the science of learning and the best practices in education and clinical practice?
5. What do you know about the Institute of Medicine reports on quality healthcare?

Overheard: *Why do we have to know theory...*

Theory is key to guiding teaching with technology. At a time when it is hard to keep up with rapidly changing technology, theories provide direction for teaching and learning. Time-tested classics, such as adult education theory, meld well with today's technology-rich environment. Theories and models serve as guides in organizing teaching and learning. They can guide our thinking and help us name more easily what we are doing. They can provide consistency or stability for faculty as they move forward with new content or new technologies.

The constant foundation of educational theories stands in contrast to constantly changing technology. This stability is encouraging because, although the content being taught and the technologies used to teach it constantly change, the theoretical underpinnings of how to teach and why to teach that way does generally not change quickly or dramatically.

Consider, for example, the question of how to teach range of motion. We know that, based on learning theories, the learning process is facilitated by students' active participation in the process. It does not matter if they participate in person, through a computer program, or via a virtual game; as long as they are actively involved, students likely learn more quickly and better remember what they have learned. The basic theoretical principle of active participation by the learner is unchanged, no matter what latest technologies are used to teach range of motion.

The best teaching and learning practices are guided by theory. In this respect, theories serve several purposes: They provide a structure or framework for teaching activities; they provide an explanation for why content is taught the way it is taught; and they often raise questions or identify issues that, without the framework, might be completely missed or ignored. Whether consciously acknowledged or not, theories help us teach well.

THEORIES: WHAT THEY ARE AND WHAT THEY ARE NOT

Theory refers to the structuring of ideas in creative and rigorous ways to "project a tentative, purposeful, and systematic view of phenomena" (Chinn & Kramer, 2011, p. 185). In our case, when we insert the word *teaching* or *learning* in place of the word *phenomena,* we see that theories provide a means of structuring ideas about teaching (or learning) in a systematic way. Well-developed theories tell us what to do and why to do it.

The application of theories to explain and justify actions is a hallmark of a profession. As educators, we use not only teaching and learning theories, but also a variety of other theories (e.g., motivational, change, team, and developmental theories). Just as important as the structure they provide, theories provide a comprehensive perspective that not only makes questions and concerns more obvious, but also provides a context in which to address them.

Any discussion of theory is fraught with the issues of semantics. What, for example, is the difference between a model and a theory? Models are simply representations of reality, and to that extent, they often are not as well developed, and their concepts and their relationships are not as well defined, as theories. However, for our purposes, the terms theory and model are used interchangeably.

Also, what is the difference between teaching, learning, and educational theories? Although there may be legitimate nuances to the connoisseur, in this book we are more concerned about the practicality of theories in supporting teaching endeavors. For example, the teaching process is facilitated by motivation among students, suggesting that teaching and learning theories alone are not enough. Rather, teaching is enhanced by the simultaneous use of motivational—and other—models and theories.

TEACHING AND LEARNING THEORIES

Many classic teaching and learning theories provide the theoretical basis of most educational texts. A brief background can be gained by considering the following classics, which are referenced frequently in the literature:

- Behaviorists believe that all behavior is learned through a fairly passive process of conditioning. Knowledge and skills that receive positive rewards are likely acquired, and those that receive negative reinforcement are likely rejected.
- Social learning theory suggests that the learning process consists of interactions among learners, their environment, and the desired knowledge and/or behavior. Observing others in the desired behavior may provide an environmental motivation to learn it. It may also help the learner see the importance of the new knowledge, which may provide the motivation necessary to learn the behavior.
- Humanistic learning theory assumes that each person is a unique individual who deserves respect, freedom, and worth and who has the desire to grow. It emphasizes individual rights, creativity, and spontaneity and suggests that learning is driven by people's subjective needs.

Three theories provide many of the basic tenants of good teaching with technologies today. A summary of each is provided with additional recommended readings. These three theories are adult learning theory, constructivist theory, and complexity theory.

Adult Learning Theory

Referred to as *andragogy* (vs. *pedagogy*, which refers to the education of children but is often used as the more common umbrella term), adult education theory is based largely on the work of Knowles (1980). Adult learners are self-directed and practical and build on experience. Their motivation generally has an internal source. They need their life experiences and accumulated knowledge base to be acknowledged, respected, and used. They learn best when they see the immediate relevance and practical application of what they are learning. Many adult learners juggle multiple responsibilities, which can create barriers to education, such as lack of time and money, scheduling problems, and childcare issues. Despite these barriers, adult learners are motivated by opportunities for personal advancement, social relationships, and a general desire for their own growth. Adult education theory reminds faculty to build on students' previous learning, engage students with the content, and use active, relevant assignments.

Constructivism Theory

Constructivism emerged from the cognitive learning theory and recognizes the past knowledge and experience of learners. Learners use prior knowledge and experience to actively build new knowledge. A pervasive tenet of constructivism is the active nature of learning, from creating the learning environment to participating in learning activities and interacting with peers and faculty. This theory emphasizes the active and autonomous role of students and defines the role of faculty in terms of facilitating that active learning process. Constructivism reminds faculty that students construct their own understandings of concepts on the basis of the content resources and tools provided.

Complexity Theory

Complexity theory provides a way to consider teaching and learning from a nonlinear perspective. Complexity theory focuses on an entire system and the underlying self-organization that occurs among the interconnections of its many individual units (Zimmerman, Plsek, & Lindberg, 2008). Nursing education requires complex learning and takes place in complex clinical situations, so this theory is often relevant to our teaching and learning considerations.

Assumptions

All theories come with their own basic assumptions. These assumptions typically lay the groundwork for how concepts are defined and how the theory's concepts relate to one another. Recognizing the assumptions of different theories provides direction in determining which theories best fit a given situation and purpose. A clinical laboratory on dressing changes provides an example. With the adult education theory, faculty are reminded to build on students' current levels of information (based on assessment), provide relevant information specific to students' learning needs, and provide an active assignment that engages students in practicing dressing changes. These adult learning principles assume that as people age and mature, they accumulate experiences that serve as a basis for future learning, as well as a readiness and desire to learn more.

ADDITIONAL THEORIES THAT SUPPLEMENT EDUCATIONAL THEORIES

Teaching and learning do not occur in isolation, so there are a variety of additional models and theories that influence the teaching and learning process. For example, education occurs within larger organizational systems, so systems theory is important. We are also concerned with the quality of education and its continued improvement, making quality-improvement theories relevant to our work, as well as the leadership necessary to guide that work. In addition, legal and ethical frameworks have gained renewed attention as technology pushes the boundaries of acceptable practice.

Systems Theories

Education generally occurs within a broader context than just the teaching and learning situation itself. For our purposes, the teaching and learning enterprise may occur within the context of a larger college or university setting that is composed of many different, but interdependent, parts. Systems theory recognizes the parts as separate and having their own responsibilities, but they are also interrelated to the overall functioning of the whole organization. One pertinent aspect of systems theory is how the organization itself operates. For example, the processes that an organization uses to change from one learning management system (LMS) to another likely includes faculty, information technology (IT), and the finance department all functioning together to make the best overall decision for students, faculty, and the institution itself. In some organizations, these processes may run very smoothly, whereas in other systems, they may not. Another pertinent aspect of systems theory is how the organization interacts with its external environment. For example, what is the impact and response of a particular campus—its IT department, faculty, and students—when the overall university system changes from one LMS to another?

Quality-Improvement Theories

Educators want to provide an excellent education so that future healthcare providers practice safely and provide quality care. Although we may already be doing a good job, we can always get better. Several different quality-improvement theories (U.S. Department of Health and Human Services, 2011) include FADE (focus, analyze, develop, execute and evaluate), PDSA (plan, do, study, and act), and Six Sigma, which consist of two different models. The two Six Sigma models include, what is referred to as DMAIC (define, measure, analyze, improve, and control) and DMADV (define, measure, analyze, design, and verify). All these models provide guidance as we aim to improve the quality of education provided to students.

Leadership Theories

Although there are a variety of leadership styles (Bradley University, 2016), transformational leadership has several components that tend to resonate within education and healthcare today. Transformational leaders use several essential components to improve outcomes and satisfaction: intellectual stimulation, individualized consideration, inspirational motivation, and idealized influence (Fischer, 2017a). Fischer (2017b) suggests that transformational leadership may decrease incivility, enhance academic–clinical relationships, and increase faculty retention.

Legal/Ethical Frameworks

Moral theories help provide guidance and ethical justification for actions taken when teaching, and both the passage of time and the advent of technology have changed education's moral landscape. Gone are the days when faculty can post grades in hard copy format outside their classroom, with students listed by name and/or student number. Not only would the names and/or student numbers be deemed inappropriate in today's environment (they would breach student privacy/confidentiality by providing identifiable information), but also when teaching with technology, the faculty may likely not have a physical classroom outside which to post the grades. Moral frameworks help educators navigate contemporary concerns ranging from confidentiality and copyright and intellectual property to newer topics such as netiquette and social spaces. Four commonly recognized ethical principles include autonomy (to respect other's choices and dignity), beneficence (to do good), nonmaleficence (to prevent or minimize harm), and justice (to treat others fairly). Other important ethical principles are privacy and confidentiality, which refer to the sharing of personal information and the way that others handle that information once it has been shared.

The Family Educational Rights and Privacy Act (FERPA) is an excellent example of the fact that although these ethical guidelines provide moral direction, their implementation must be supported by consistent policies, procedures, and legislation. FERPA is a federal law that was passed to protect the privacy of students' educational records (Hlavac, G. C., & Easterly, E. J., 2015). The law requires all institutions receiving federal funds to follow certain procedures when disclosing protected information about educational records to a third party, regardless of how that information is transmitted (mail, verbal, fax, or electronic).

BEST TEACHING PRACTICES

Like theories, best practices transcend both the content being taught and the technology being used to teach it. Although there may be several ways to teach safe medication administration (on a classmate, on a patient, or on a computer-generated patient), the same basic theoretical principles and the same basic best practices apply to all methods. The science of learning refers to multidisciplinary studies that investigate how knowledge and skills are acquired and the reasons why some methods work and others do not (Kim, McGivney, & Care, 2017). Best teaching practices are strategies that are supported by science and that produce good teaching and learning outcomes. Some 30 years ago, Chickering and Gamson (1987) were early best-practice adopters, using research to identify seven principles of good teaching and learning in undergraduate education. Carnegie Mellon University subsequently expanded Chickering and Gamson's classic work on best teaching principles, which have been developed from a variety of disciplines using the best evidence available.

Carnegie Mellon University's (2015) best teaching principles are as follows: (a) Prior knowledge can help or hurt the learning process, (b) knowledge organization affects how students learn, (c) motivation supports student learning, (d) students must learn basic knowledge and ways to integrate and use those skills to achieve mastery, (e) learning is improved with focused practice and specific feedback, (f) the interaction between course environment and the student's developmental level affects learning, and (g) students need the skills to manage the ways they learn best to become self-directed learners. Bain (2004) has also contributed to this discussion about best teaching practices, emphasizing that faculty must believe that students are capable of learning and that teaching does matter, all of which is nicely summarized by the Missouri State University Faculty Center for Teaching and Learning (2017).

Bain (2012) has also written about best practices for students, reminding us how important their role is in the process. The following teaching and learning principles remain relevant today (University of Michigan, 2016):

1. Previous knowledge and experience can either help or hurt future learning.
2. Motivation creates and sustains positive learning behaviors.
3. The way learners organize knowledge affects their appropriate use of that knowledge.
4. Skills and knowledge, synthesis, and application are all necessary for content mastery.
5. Learning requires practice focused on specific goals, as well as focused feedback.
6. Self-directed learners can monitor, evaluate, and adjust their learning activities as needed.
7. Because learners are holistic beings, the social and emotional aspects of the classroom affect their learning.

An evidence-based review abstract, Learning to Learn With Concept Mapping, is shared at the end of the chapter (see Exhibit 3.2). Recognizing concepts as the principal components of theories, this systematic review explicitly combines theory and best practices and provides faculty direction for engaging students in their own learning by using orientation sessions on concept mapping.

THEORY, INSTITUTE OF MEDICINE, AND HEALTH PROFESSIONALS IMPLICATIONS

Models and theories also help organize the vast amounts of information that exist in the rapidly changing clinical world. Although this book focuses primarily on theory as a way to organize teaching activities, it is important for both faculty and students to recognize that models and theories are useful organizers for clinical content too. Randomly scattered bits of clinical information are of limited use to students and clinicians. Pulling these information bits together with a conceptual model or theory promotes an organized approach to learning and later recall of the topic. Models of pain management that address structural and functional pathophysiology and then relate it to the best pain-management evidence are some of the examples. Population-focused theories (e.g., theories on the aging or the cardiac-failure population) also help organize and generalize scattered clinical information into more cohesive frameworks that assist clinical students in learning to provide safe care based on best practices supported by the science of learning.

Knowing and using theories and best teaching practices is vital, but theory without proper content is useless. In nursing, there always seems to be too much content and too little time to teach it. Similarly, it seems as if there is always so much new content to include, yet no old content to relinquish. Using a conceptual (i.e., theoretical) approach to teaching can help faculty make difficult decisions about what really needs to be taught by organizing an overwhelming number of information bits into a more manageable framework.

Like the constantly changing teaching technologies that are the focus of this book, technology is creating fast-paced, constant change in the content of clinical practice. Consequently, technology affects the content of the clinical content taught to future healthcare clinicians. As context for this discussion, it is important to know that the Institute of Medicine (IOM) published a series of reports (see Exhibit 3.1) on varying aspects of the healthcare system in the 1990s and early 2000s with the intent of improving that very system. The number and extent of these reports indicated the need for faculty and students alike to understand and apply the principles promulgated. Further discussion regarding the import of these reports for nursing education is provided by Finkelman and Kenner (2012). Technology provides a powerful tool with which to collect, analyze, and disseminate the evidence necessary to establish these best clinical recommendations, and it is also a powerful tool by which to teach students about these recommendations.

EXHIBIT 3.1

CLASSIC IOM REPORTS SPECIFIC TO CLINICAL HEALTH PROFESSIONS EDUCATION

Each of these reports can be located online by running an Internet search for the title. A summary of IOM reports is provided by Finkelman and Kenner (2012).

SAFETY REPORTS

To Err Is Human (1999)
Patient Safety: Achieving a New Standard of Care (2004)

(continued)

QUALITY REPORTS

Crossing the Quality Chasm (2001)
Envisioning the National Healthcare Quality (2001)
Priority Areas for National Action: Transforming Healthcare Quality (2003)

LEADERSHIP REPORT

Leadership by Example: Coordinating Government Roles in Improving Healthcare Quality (2003)

PUBLIC HEALTH REPORTS

The Future of the Public's Health in the 21st Century (2003)
Who Will Keep the Public Health? (2003)
Unequal Treatment: Confronting Racial and Ethnic Disparities in Healthcare (2002)
Guidance for the National Healthcare Disparities Report (2002)

NURSING REPORT

Keeping Patients Safe: Transforming the Work Environment for Nurses (2004)

HEALTH PROFESSIONS EDUCATION REPORT

Health Professional Education: A Bridge to Quality (2003)

IOM, Institute of Medicine.

The IOM reports (Finkelman & Kenner, 2012) have identified 20 priority areas of care for evidence-based clinical practice. To ensure that clinicians are properly prepared to address these priority areas and the systems in which they work, critical curricular components are also identified. Six improvement goals relate to healthcare being safe, effective, patient-centered, timely, efficient, and equitable (IOM, 2001).

These IOM recommendations are comprehensive and far reaching. The reports demonstrate the extent to which the entire context in which healthcare providers, and nurses in particular, are educated must change to accomplish these goals. The educational implications of the IOM resources have been further discussed (Finkelman & Kenner, 2012). Technology represents a key mechanism by which best clinical practices are established, and best teaching practices facilitate their implementation through the education of both new and established practitioners. Five core competencies for health professions have been identified and their acknowledgment has been widespread. The broad concepts also provide direction for teaching with technologies. The five core competencies identified by the IOM (2003) include the following:

- Provide patient-centered care
- Work in interdisciplinary teams
- Use evidence-based practice
- Apply quality improvement
- Use informatics

INTEGRATED LEARNING TRIANGLE FOR TEACHING WITH TECHNOLOGIES

In the Integrated Learning Triangle for Teaching With Technologies (see Exhibit 1.3), both theories and best teaching practices are represented by the outer circle. They are part of the broader sphere in which a specific teaching activity is situated. Theories and best practices represent knowledge that is foundational to educational experiences in general, so they are represented by the outside circle in which any particular teaching activity and related decisions are placed.

As discussed earlier, the evidence-based review abstract, Learning to Learn With Concept Mapping, is provided in Exhibit 3.2. This synthesis of best evidence provides further direction for our work as educators.

EXHIBIT 3.2

EVIDENCE-BASED REVIEW ABSTRACT: LEARNING TO LEARN WITH CONCEPT MAPPING

Compiled by: Patricia Conejo, PhD, RN, WHNP

The following summary provides a graduate student's experience of synthesizing literature for her work using concept maps to help students learn basic nursing content.

Students need to be prepared as lifelong learners. Helping students learn to use concept maps is one strategy for promoting critical thinking and lifelong learning. Literature supports that these holistic visual representations, encourage active learning, improve critical thinking, and increase knowledge retention; students better understand patient conditions and planning of nursing care. Strategies for teaching students how best to learn with concept maps (including literature on best evidence for concept maps and guidelines for helping students learn with concept maps) were reviewed.

Recommendations for best practices drawn from the literature included providing clear instructions, using a valid and reliable rubric, and creating opportunities for reflection via peer and faculty feedback. Piloting of the best evidence with a group of students included a narrated PowerPoint presentation (Learning to Learn with Concept Maps) assignment guidelines, a feedback worksheet, and a rubric. The assignment was to draw a concept map for one of the two situations of relevance for nursing students: organization of the multiple course assignments for the semester or time management to balance the demands of work, home, and school. Student responses, including concept maps, written feedback, and in-class discussion, were evaluated for themes and evidence of critical thinking.

A major theme that emerged was student openness to trying concept mapping but not being accustomed to the nonlinear approach. The greatest challenge appeared to lie in motivating students to take the time to reorient their thinking patterns to this more holistic, big-picture approach. Further study of effective methods for moving students in this direction is needed. Students who develop their high-level thinking skills as a result of concept mapping will be better prepared for ongoing learning and care of patients in the increasingly complex and rapidly evolving environment of today's healthcare.

SUMMARY

As faculty struggle to keep up with rapidly changing content and technologies, models and theories serve as tools to help organize approaches and provide consistency and stability. Supported by the science of learning, these theories and best teaching practices provide the evidence-based guidance necessary to make teaching endeavors successful. The IOM calls for a similar process in the healthcare system, in which the best clinical practices would provide the guidance necessary for good clinical outcomes. As these best clinical practices emerge, technologies provide teaching platforms for disseminating information to students and healthcare providers.

ENDING REFLECTIONS FOR YOUR LEARNING NOTEBOOK

1. What is the most important content that you learned in this chapter?
2. What are your plans for using the information in this chapter in your future teaching endeavors?
3. What are your further learning goals?

GUIDELINES FOR THEORY AND TEACHING TECHNOLOGIES

Quick Teaching Tips

1. Choose teaching and learning theories that best fit a particular course or content and student learners.
2. Actively engage students in the content you're teaching as often as possible.
3. Include emphasis in all classes on the health professions' core competencies: patient-centered care, interdisciplinary teams, evidence-based practice, quality improvement, and informatics.

Questions for Further Reflection

1. How do theory, technology, and clinical teaching principles mesh to create quality healthcare in the future?
2. What are the implications of theory, technology, and best practices on your own self-directed, lifelong learning practices?

Learning Activity: Introductory Letter to Students

This learning activity will help instructors reflect on the theories they use when teaching and articulate their reasons for doing using them.

How does adult education theory (or another theory) help you think about your own approach to teaching and learning? Are the concepts similar or different from your plans for working with students in a technology-rich setting? Imagine that you have an opportunity to share your theory of education in the form of a letter to current (or future) students for a specific class you will teach. Write an introductory letter to students about your class, sharing your approaches to teaching and learning. Include comments about how technology will be used in your class. As you write your letter, what aspects of adult education (or other) theory guide you?

Learning Activity: Theory Contest

The purpose of this learning activity is to help students realize exactly how dependent their teaching and/or clinical practice is on a broad theoretical base. Milliken and Grace (2017) suggest that nurses need to be willing and able to recognize the ethical nature of their practice before they can act as moral agents. Similarly, we suggest that students and nurses must also be aware of the theoretical nature of their practice before they can consciously identify the theories that guide their practice and the power those theories provide.

This contest has several variations (use your imagination and creativity) and is applicable to any teaching situation or patient population (e.g., pediatric cardiology). One variation is to have students write down as many theories that apply to their care of a pediatric cardiology patient as they can think of. After the set amount of time, students start sharing their theories as you compile a master list that is visible to all students. When students think they are done, you ask for three more applicable theories. Again, when students think they are done, ask for three more theories. No repeats are allowed; if the theory is questionable, rationale may be requested. Be sure to provide time and not rush because this exercise is difficult at the beginning, and student groups may take time to catch on and generate a long list of appropriate theories—an eye-opening experience for increasing the awareness of students who initially do not see the direct applicability of theory.

Online Resources for Further Learning

- University of Michigan, Center for Research on Learning and Teaching. This site contains an index of educational theories, as well as links to additional theory sites: www.crlt.umich.edu/tstrategies/tslt
- National League for Nursing. This site describes hallmarks of outstanding education, including categories such as students, faculty, curriculum, and teaching and valuation strategies: www.nln.org/professional-development -programs/teaching-resources/excellence-model

REFERENCES

Bain, K. (2004). *What the best college teachers do*. Cambridge, MA: President and Fellows of Harvard College.

Bain, K. (2012). *What the best college students do*. Cambridge, MA: President and Follows of Harvard College.

Bradley University. (2016). How nursing leadership styles can impact patient outcomes and organizational performance. Retrieved from http://onlinedegrees.bradley.edu/resources/infographics/how-nursing-leadership-styles-can-impact-patient-outcomes-and-organizational-performance

Carnegie Mellon University. (2015). Theory and research-based principles of learning. Retrieved from https://www.cmu.edu/teaching/principles/learning.html

Chickering, A. W., & Gamson, Z. F. (1987). Seven principles for good practice in undergraduate education. Retrieved from https://files.eric.ed.gov/fulltext/ED282491.pdf

Chinn, P. L., & Kramer, M. K. (2011). *Integrated theory and knowledge development in nursing* (8th ed.). St Louis, MO: Elsevier Mosby.

Finkelman, A., & Kenner, C. (2012). *Teaching IOM: Implications of the Institute of Medicine reports for nursing education* (3rd ed.). Silver Spring, MD: American Nurses Association.

Fischer, S. A. (2017a). Developing nurses' transformational leadership skills. *Nursing Standard, 31*(51), 54–63. doi:10.7748/ns.2017.e10857

Fischer, S. A. (2017b). Transformational leadership in nursing education. *Nursing Science Quarterly, 30*(2):124–128. doi:10.1177/0894318417693309

Hlavac, G. C., & Easterly, E. J. (2015). FERPA primer: The basics and beyond. Retrieved from http://www.naceweb.org/public-policy-and-legal/legal-issues/ferpa-primer-the-basics-and-beyond

Institute of Medicine. (2001). *Crossing the quality chasm*. Washington, DC: National Academies Press.

Institute of Medicine. (2003). *Health professions education: A bridge to quality*. Washington, DC: National Academies Press.

Kim, H., McGivney, E., & Care, E. (2017). Science of learning: Why do we care? *Brookings Institution*. Retrieved from https://www.brookings.edu/blog/education-plus-development/2017/03/28/science-of-learning-why-do-we-care

Knowles, M. S. (1980). *The modern practice of adult education. From pedagogy to andragogy* (2nd ed.). Englewood Cliffs, NJ: Prentice Hall.

Milliken, A., & Grace, P. (2017). Nurse ethical awareness: Understanding the nature of everyday practice. *Nursing Ethics, 24*(5), 517–524. doi:10.1177/0969733015615172

Missouri State University Faculty Center for Teaching and Learning. (2017). Best practices for teaching and learning. Retrieved from https://www.missouristate.edu/fctl/89072.htm

United States Department of Health and Human Services, Health Resources and Services Administration. (2011). Quality Improvement. Retrieved from https://www.hrsa.gov/sites/default/files/quality/toolbox/pdfs/qualityimprovement.pdf

University of Michigan. (2016). Research-based principles of learning & teaching strategies. Retrieved from http://www.crlt.umich.edu/print/19716

Zimmerman, B., Plsek, P., & Lindberg, C. (2008). *Edgeware: Insights from complexity science for health care leaders*. Irving, TX: Plexus Institute.

CHAPTER 4

Technology Teaching and Learning: Engaging Assignments and Lesson Plans

CHAPTER GOAL

Gain practical tips for translating course content into instructional form, using lesson plans and engaging assignments to focus the use of technologies.

BEGINNING REFLECTION

1. How would you rate your experiences and comfort with writing lesson plans?
2. Are you comfortable in helping students prepare for class, leading them through class, and then challenging them to use the materials after leaving class?
3. How will you use technologies to engage students in learning?

Overheard: *Aren't lesson plans a tool of the past? Shouldn't we just be spontaneous in presenting our classes?*

This chapter is about organizing a plan to make technology an efficient part of our teaching and our students' learning outcomes. Why does the lesson plan help us make sense of our work in teaching with technologies? Technology does not solve all teaching problems, but particularly with a new generation of student learners, it may provide useful tools for engaging students in learning. Lesson plans help us think about and choose reasonable options for using technology to accomplish learning purposes. Lesson plans provide a thoughtful approach to our teaching and can help us decide when and whether technologies enhance learning. Lesson plans make teaching more than a random act; they can make teaching a purposeful activity that can be evaluated and developed further over time.

LESSON PLANS AS ORGANIZING TOOLS

A lesson plan is considered a guide for teaching and learning plans. Lesson plans come in many shapes and sizes, but in almost all cases, they influence our classroom accomplishments. If we don't use a road map to determine where we are going with our teaching and learning plans, we may not reach our destination efficiently and effectively. Lesson plans provide a way of capturing and organizing our content and our plans for helping students learn (Nilson, 2016). Many components go into lesson planning, and these components provide ways to organize ideas into meaningful classes. Although lesson plans provide the written, organized format for a class, technology supplies the hands-on, doing approach to teaching and learning. It is important to put technology into the lesson plan only when it provides the best learning. Lesson plans provide direction for a class and remind us why and how technology will be used to accomplish class objectives.

Lesson plans are a way to organize our thinking, helping us choose from among a variety of options for teaching a concept. Technology can promote efficiency and effectiveness in considering and organizing materials. For example, in how many ways can diabetic foot care be taught? What are the best approaches for a particular student group? The Learning Activity in this chapter outlines some ideas for thinking about this process. As we begin the diabetic foot care exercise, it is essential to think about: who are the learners; what are their particular learning needs related to diabetic foot care; how best to accomplish the teaching and learning activity; whether a selected technology will be useful; and what the anticipated outcomes should be.

INTEGRATED LEARNING TRIANGLE FOR TEACHING WITH TECHNOLOGIES AS A GUIDE

Lesson plans help organize our classes. The Integrated Learning Triangle for Teaching With Technologies (see Exhibit 1.3) provides direction, helping us make the best choices among the many ways that content can be taught. For example, if faculty are preparing to teach a class on wound care, they may consider in many ways it can be taught and ways that technology can be included. Wound care lectures, videos, clinical laboratories, and review of websites or readings about wound care with electronic quizzes are examples of some of the many ways to teach. All these clearly provide learning opportunities, but we as faculty, as well as students, all have finite amounts of time to accomplish our learning purposes. Choosing the best learning options for a given context is what lesson plans help us do. The Integrated Learning Triangle for Teaching With Technologies is one tool for further developing our technology-supported lesson plans.

In applying the Integrated Learning Triangle for Teaching With Technologies in lesson plan development, it is initially important to consider the context. Because all nursing classes are different, the logistics, resources, and context remind us to focus on who our learners are, what resources are available for teaching and learning (including time frames, people resources, and technologies), and what the needed learning outcomes are. Context also reminds us to set a particular course within the context of a course curriculum (building on prior learning and creating a path to further learning in future classes).

Other points of the Integrated Learning Triangle for Teaching With Technologies remind us to assess where learners are (related to the content), what their needed learning outcomes are, what teaching and learning activities might best help them achieve learning, what is the best fit for technology applications, what feedback is needed to keep learning on track, and, ultimately, what is needed to build quality improvement into daily lesson planning. In wound care, for example, basic considerations include leveling student learning needs from beginning to more advanced, determining wound types and wound care procedures from simple to more complex, and deciphering the type of learning activities that might best fit this intended lesson plan given this context. This might include, for example, engaging technologies such as active simulations or virtual reality scenarios.

FORMAT FOR LESSON PLANS

Organizing the content for a lesson plan is sometimes challenging, given the myriad of content that exists in nursing. Diverse formats can be used for communicating lesson plans because there is not only one right way. A template approach to course and lesson planning that begins with the desired outcomes and works backward to objectives and learning activities can be used (Wiggins & McTighe, 2006). Others use an outline format as the easiest way to summarize a lesson plan. A one-page visual class organizer can serve as both a lesson plan and a communication tool. For example, you will want the lesson plan to be specific enough that others would know what should be covered, what strategies to use to do the teaching (including use of technologies), and how to evaluate learning outcomes. Often, one specific, school-wide, lesson plan format is developed by a faculty team. In rapidly changing clinical arenas, complexity theory supports that broad questions guide us in determining content to be considered (Zimmerman, Plsek, Lindberg, 2008).

Once student learning needs are identified, a lesson plan can be built. Thinking about the lesson plan as a communication tool (for yourself and others) provides direction in plan development. A lesson plan-commonly includes the following categories:

- Objectives/outcome statements
- Organization of "must-know" content or concepts
- Active teaching and learning plans (including appropriate technologies) to engage learners
- Assessments with time allotments

- Evaluation and feedback plans
- Review and revisions

OBJECTIVES AND OUTCOME STATEMENTS AS LESSON PLAN ORGANIZERS

Learning objectives and outcome statements serve as key tools in lesson plans (Nilson, 2016). In recent years, outcome-based education has been emphasized, further stressing that students need to be clearly informed early on about assessment criteria (Keating, 2015). Objectives are more specific than outcomes: They are delineated with educational domains (cognitive/knowledge, affective/attitudes, or psychomotor/skills); composed with verbs to observe, measure, and assess; and used to guide the teaching and learning experience for the teacher and student. In comparison, outcomes identify the behaviors that define and signify the achievement of objectives. Outcomes validate the evidence that a teacher will accept, which means a student has achieved the objective (Nilson, 2016). Outcomes relate directly to professional practice. Outcomes can be defined from foundational, to remediating, to ultimate program learning outcomes. It is important for each school to define objectives and outcomes with clarity and consistency within the curriculum.

Just as there are many different types of picture frames (each varied picture frame showcasing the picture in a different way), there are many ways to frame a lesson (and many ways to incorporate technologies into the lesson plan). A teacher must remember to develop the lesson plan using a systematic process that delineates objectives from implementation through evaluation of the teaching and learning experience.

A clearly written objective is vital for evaluating the learner-focused assessment, including characteristics of ABCD: audience or the learners, behavior or performance that will be expected and how it will be measured using a domain (cognitive/knowledge, psychomotor/skill, and affective/attitude), conditions that the learner is expected to use to perform the behavior, and degree or criterion to which the behavior is to be evaluated.

Objectives should be learner focused and composed at an appropriate student learning level; this means that objectives are not too narrowly developed, making them difficult to manage, and conversely, are not so general that they provide little guidance for instruction. Objectives are determined based on student characteristics and needs and vary based on the educational level of students and the way that the content is presented. Once determined, they provide the framework for creating appropriate teaching and learning strategies based on best teaching evidence.

Bloom's (1956) taxonomy is a well-known resource for developing instructional objectives with leveling for students. A taxonomy is a classification system that describes and identifies using the three domains of learning (cognitive/ knowledge, affective/attitude, and psychomotor/skill). Bloom's taxonomy has hierarchical levels of learning, from lowest to highest: knowledge, comprehension, application, analysis, synthesis, and evaluation. The taxonomy originally referred to the cognitive/knowledge domain, but subsequent editions also dealt with affective and psychomotor learning domains. Anderson and Krathwohl (2001) published revised terminology for Bloom's taxonomy. Most notably, the authors amended Bloom's taxonomy processes from nouns to verbs, and the highest hierarchical category was changed to "create." An Internet search on these taxonomies can help you identify guides to use in developing and evaluating objectives. In addition, see Exhibit 4.1 for a self-assessment for evaluating written objectives.

A commonly used acronym framework when finalizing well-written objectives for lesson plans is **SMART** (Wayne State University, 2017). SMART objectives are specific, measurable, acceptable to the instructor, realistic, and time bound. Specific details what task will occur; measurement defines the accuracy of evaluation using a performance standard; acceptable defines the indicators that determine task completion by the instructor; realism asks if the task can be done given the setting and resources; and time-orientated answers when the task is to be completed. It is important to realize that tasks commonly build on one another (referred to as scaffolding) and can be interrelated concepts for educational milestones (Nilson, 2016). Milestones help students and teachers periodically assess learning outcomes, which is important for the development of continued learning opportunities that validate successful completion of leveled performance expectations.

Assignments that capture technology for additional study are presented in graphic form in the Modern Taxonomy Wheel. In an effort to help educators better integrate technology into meaningful teaching and learning, the Modern

EXHIBIT 4.1

SELF-ASSESSMENT TO EVALUATE WRITTEN OBJECTIVES

When objectives are written, a few things to self-assess against, include the following. Ask yourself if you were able to:

- Keep objectives specific enough to measure but broad enough to allow some flexibility in the class?
- Make your objectives as action oriented as possible and as high a level in Bloom's taxonomy as appropriate for your learner's level?
- Include affective verbs such as *value* and *appreciate*?
- Include objectives that allow students to complete the three domains of learning: cognitive/knowledge, psychomotor/skill, and affective/attitude?
- Consider the ABCD characteristics of well-written objectives?
- Analyze objectives using the SMART format: Is the objective specific, measurable, acceptable to the instructor, realistic to achieve, and time bound?

Taxonomy Wheel was generated by Allan Carrington (Kharbach, 2017). This wheel is a visually stimulating tool that integrates Bloom's taxonomies with action verbs, activities, and suggested technologies for lesson plans. As Raman (2015) explains, mobile technology needs to be enhanced in the classroom, clinical, and laboratory settings using structured activities, assessments, evaluations, and faculty role modeling. The Modern Taxonomy Wheel is available online and is a suggested tool for synthesizing mobile technology into nursing education for engaging assignments (see Online Resources for Further Learning at chapter end).

CLARIFYING AND ORGANIZING THE "MUST-KNOW" CONTENT

How much content is too much? How much is enough? At a time of "information overload," faculty can avoid trying to teach everything in the books by focusing on the "must-know" concepts for specified classes. A national dialogue on organization of learning materials via broad concepts supports helping students learn conceptually with exemplars versus trying to memorize long laundry lists of information. Again, the advent of smartphones and quickly accessible information provides students fingertip access to detailed points of unusual disease symptoms or medication interactions.

The rapid advances in clinical knowledge also challenge faculty to stay updated on the breadth of subjects being taught. The faculty role in being knowledgeable in practice and maintaining content competence is even considered an ethical issue (American Association for Higher Education, 1993; National League for Nursing, 2013). The advent of technologies supports faculty work in being seekers of information and equally important, role modeling this to students.

As noted, thinking about content and objectives go hand in hand. Adult education reminds us to focus on what the learners need to know relevant to their current or future practice (Knowles, 1984). Guides for how to make presentations clear are summarized by McKeachie and Svinicki (2014) and suggest beginning with simple, familiar concepts; using multiple examples; and eliminating nonessential information. Simple ways to begin organization can be facilitated with technology such as electronic concept maps and organizers. In addition, consider the following points:

- Emphasize key points via concepts that are initially broad and allow application to diverse populations; further detail can then build on these broad concepts.
- Keep material manageable (the key points) and logically organized.
- Use the "chunking" approach to organize information (breaking up long streams of information into manageable units to improve recall).

If we start with the basics or the main concepts to be covered, helping the learner understand why these key points or concepts are important, we can then build more specific information onto that base. Furthermore, grouping like information can help recall. For example, you might have a learning objective to help students understand the broad concept of anti-inflammatory drugs. Rather than having students try to outline and memorize each specific drug, focus on the broader class of drugs (a type of "chunking").

Also, appropriate questions can help guide our thinking about lesson planning, focusing on learning needs. For example, beginning questions specific to the learners' needs incorporates the cognitive (knowledge), psychomotor (skill), and affective (attitude) learning domains:

1. Cognitive: What specific facts are needed?
2. Psychomotor: What specific skills are needed?
3. Affective: What values or attitudes are needed?

In using these questions (e.g., in a class about strategies to promote older adults' self-care for medication management), students need to appreciate that promoting self-care is important (affective) and that simple strategies (such as cueing techniques) can promote older adults' self-care (cognitive). Finally, students should be able to demonstrate self-care–promotion strategies in their work with patients (psychomotor).

ADDITIONAL CONSIDERATIONS: PRECLASS AND POSTCLASS LEARNING AND TECHNOLOGIES

Preclass and postclass learning activities in our lesson plans support and encourage significant learning (Fink, 2013). The concept of creating both "set" and "closure" helps capture these ideas within a lesson plan. Technology then provides opportunities for additional assignments, helping students capture further details or nice-to-know information beyond the classroom.

Creating Set for a Class Session or Presentation

Set, just like it sounds, includes setting the stage for learning. Set includes helping students prepare for class (e.g., preclass assignments) and then setting a positive tone for learning once students arrive in class. Technology has enhanced our opportunities for supporting students' preparation for class. Students can electronically submit items, such as learning quizzes, key points from readings, or brief paragraphs about their experiences, with a topic before class begins. The first few minutes of your class time (or introductory materials if online) sets the stage for learning. Examples include synthesizing points from student preclass submissions, sharing a story about the topic to engage their interest, and highlighting the major points to be gained from the presentation. Clickers or automated response systems also support opportunities for in-class learning quizzes based on assigned readings.

Creating Closure for a Class or Presentation

Closure, just like it sounds, involves getting the most from the closing minutes of your class or from closing communications if online). This step includes strategies such as "summaries" and review questions and provides the opportunity to reinforce content one last time. Fink (2013) recommends using this time to challenge students to use the information gained, as well as to help students set further learning goals. In a classroom, this step might include setting aside the last 10 minutes of class to use reinforcement strategies. In an online class, this "what next" step might be conveyed through a final summary of module activity. In a clinical practicum, this step may involve reflecting on best patient care practices with student interventions in postconference and in clinical journals. This can also remind students of further learning resources for opportunities to expand learning.

ACTIVE LEARNING AND TECHNOLOGY TO ENGAGE THE LEARNER

Once we have identified the objectives, there are numerous ways to achieve them. Our goal is to enhance our skills at providing content to students in ways that help them understand, remember, and apply the information. Complexity theory (Zimmerman et al, 2008) reminds us of the numerous pathways and processes for students to gain successful learning outcomes.

Using a variety of interactive teaching strategies helps meet the needs of a diverse audience. Bean (2011) summarizes a variety of tools that serve as assignments in engaging students in active learning and that include ideas for active writing assignments and problem-based learning. A combination of teaching strategies keeps presentations interesting and perhaps even fun. An interactive component promotes students' participation in learning. Remembering basic educational principles helps direct the following combinations of learning approaches (many based on technologies) to best fit your learners' needs.

- ■ *Verbal or audio strategies.* Use lecture judiciously as an important tool for conveying selected facts. Incorporate questions for thought or discussion into lectures to promote interest and increase their effectiveness. The addition of storytelling can bridge practice and theory. For example, in a lecture on self-care, briefly describe the specific techniques that can be used to promote self-care and then share a story or case example. Then build in questions that help students frame and solve problems using the story or case as background information related to challenges and approaches for promoting self-care.
- ■ *Visual strategies.* Provide multiple sensory cues about a topic, such as adding a visual component to the spoken word, to promote students' understanding and retention of information. Using imagery techniques helps students understand why the topic is important for patients. It is often helpful to build on basic strategies of "watching" or observing a technique or process, whether by video or in real time. Technology is at our fingertips.

■ ***Kinesthetic or doing strategies.*** Individuals often learn best by doing; practice can enhance the link between the facts presented and the actual clinical application of those facts. Role playing or simulations can be a warm-up for the clinical practice experience or an alternate approach when actual supervised practice is not practical. Supervised practice in a learning laboratory setting or a clinical setting promotes the opportunity to check off learning competencies. In addition, arranging student observations with peer review is a key lifelong learning strategy.

The activities noted—auditory, visual, and doing strategies—can be used with technologies to further develop a lesson plan. A variety of interactive strategies, such as discussion questions, case study, and role-play, can be used to promote the practice and retention of materials. Another approach includes using the mnemonic FIRE (focused program content, interactive teaching methods, reinforced learning, and evaluation) to guide lesson planning (see Exhibit 4.2). When this tool is used, a variety of adult education principles for promoting teaching and learning are incorporated into a class session.

As we consider basic presentation plans, we think about our use of active learning strategies that promote student engagement and critical thinking. A variety of interactive strategies, such as discussion questions, case study, and role playing, can be used to promote the practice and retention of materials. A resource with further examples is the Quality and Safety Education for Nurses Institute (QSEN, 2017) modules designed to engage new and experienced faculty. These QSEN modules, including topics such as informatics and simulation, integrate quality and safety competencies using a variety of teaching methods that engage users.

EVALUATION AND FEEDBACK

Assignment blueprints and evaluation templates are keys to a successful class. According to Walvoord, Anderson, and Angelo (2009), what students have to do to earn an A should be the same as what they have to do to learn well. This

---

EXHIBIT 4.2

FIRED-UP TEACHING

Use the following concepts to light a **FIRE** for your class teaching:

Focused program content: Emphasize key points and make content relevant and easily applicable.

Interactive teaching strategies: Use a variety of strategies to meet the needs of diverse audiences.

Reinforced learning: Share information repeatedly from a variety of perspectives.

Evaluated learning: Help students reflect and identify what they have learned.

concept works in guiding both teaching practices and evaluation. In Chapter 9, evaluation concepts are discussed in more detail. Strategies for developing an assignment and evaluation blueprint based on lesson plan objectives/outcomes are also discussed. Concepts for evaluating key points or a "fired-up" lesson plan are provided in Exhibit 4.2.

Consistent with our discussion of preparing students for learning, the evidence based review abstract "Best Practices for Orienting Students to Learning" is provided in Exhibit 4.3. This synthesis of best evidence provides further direction for our work as educators.

EXHIBIT 4.3

EVIDENCE-BASED REVIEW ABSTRACT: BEST PRACTICE FOR ORIENTING STUDENTS TO LEARNING

Compiled by: Suzanne Stricklin, PhD, RN, CNE

The following summary provides a graduate student's experience conducting an evidence-based review on the topic of orientating students to learning.

The Challenge. Much of course and clinical orientation for undergraduate nursing students is rote in nature and of little use. Several hours of class time and entire clinical days are spent on this topic, yet students do not feel as if their questions have been answered. Instead, many feel overwhelmed and believe that the instructor is asking the impossible. Learning takes on new and exciting avenues every day, yet our orientations have not followed. Students are crying for assistance in how to sort through the extensive amount of information presented, but little time is used in addressing such issues. The purpose of this abstract is to establish a framework for student orientation that allows for maintaining high expectations and excellence while giving students what they need to be successful.

Synthesis/Interpretation of Literature. Although limited literature exists on this topic, findings include the following: (a) Exercises geared toward specific course objectives are helpful when new areas are being introduced; (b) specific high-risk groups may need additional orientation geared to their particular needs; (c) anxiety may be a useful topic (especially test anxiety) to address; (d) students want communication with peers and faculty that is not just cursory; (e) most of the administrative information should be left out and given in another way); (f) use of "mastery-oriented teaching practices" when introducing material promotes increased persistence; (g) when faculty are introduced, encouragement of help-seeking is essential and needs to be followed up on regularly thereafter; (h) introduction of specific study strategies may increase success; (i) week-long orientations may promote success in some populations; (j) the same material should not be presented in each class because the students get bored quickly and tune you out; and (k) students want substantive content early.

Brief Model Case. Application of this evidence could be accomplished by providing new faculty an opportunity to assess their current personal knowledge, followed by exploring best practice in orienting students. They could be asked to gather previously used orientation plans/materials or develop a list of items they believe should be included in the orientation of a course they are teaching in the upcoming semester, including who, what, when, where, how, and why factors. After presentation of the evidence, faculty could be asked to rethink their orientation plans and to identify specific changes they will make based on the evidence.

SUMMARY

Using lesson plans to organize classes can remind us to make technology an efficient part of our teaching and our students' learning outcomes. The lesson plan structure provides direction and guidance in preparing effective classes. Lesson plans incorporate objectives/outcomes, "must-know" content, active learning assignments, and evaluation plans using appropriate technologies to engage the learners.

ENDING REFLECTIONS FOR YOUR LEARNING NOTEBOOK

1. What is the most important content you gained from this chapter?
2. What plan do you have for putting this information into action?
3. What are your further learning goals?

GUIDELINES FOR TEACHING AND LEARNING WITH TECHNOLOGIES

Quick Teaching Tips

1. Package the lesson plan in a way that others can use and learn from (meaning the plan can serve from semester to semester).
2. Use the Integrated Learning Triangle for Teaching With Technologies to help organize a class session or module.
3. Assimilate a variety of assignment types to engage diverse learners.
4. Gain input and critique from colleagues.

Questions for Further Reflection

1. What is the role of lesson plans in preparing health professions students of the future?
2. What ways can technology be used to promote engaging assignments?

Learning Activity: Create a Lesson Plan

HOW MANY WAYS ARE THERE TO TEACH DIABETIC FOOT CARE?

The purpose of this learning activity is to practice developing a lesson plan. A suggested topic for this lesson plan activity is teaching diabetic foot care. As you develop this assignment, apply the Integrated Learning Triangle for Teaching With Technologies (see Exhibit 1.3) to guide best choices among the many ways that content can be taught and incorporate common lesson plan categories explained in this chapter. Complete this activity using the checklist to self-assess lesson plans (see Exhibit 4.4).

EXHIBIT 4.4

LESSON PLAN SELF-ASSESSMENT CHECKLIST

A few self-assessment points to consider when developing lesson plans follow. Have you considered the following?

1. Assessing your learners' differing needs, learning styles, and knowledge backgrounds?
2. Stating specific objectives/outcomes (even though there are multiple ways to meet them)?
3. Organizing the "must-know" content in a reasonable outline format?
4. Enhancing motivations to learn by creating set and learning incentives?
5. Asking learners to prepare and actively participate in your classes?
6. Using multiple approaches to enhance learning?
7. Incorporating evaluation into your lesson plan?
8. Enhancing the use of information presented with closure strategies that include reflecting on what has been learned and the ways that it might be applied in the future?

Consider the following questions as you think about the components to your diabetic foot care lesson plan:

- Should all classes on diabetic foot care be taught the same way?
- Is technology required to teach this topic?
- Could selected technologies enhance learning?
- Are students best taught by watching a video? By listening to a podcast? By demonstration and practice?
- How can you incorporate strategies that encourage critical thinking about diabetic foot care?
- What evaluation strategies will you use to document diabetic foot care learning?
- How many possible ways can you identify to teach this content and develop your lesson plan?

Online Resources for Further Learning

- Arizona State University (2017) Teach Online. This resource provides teaching resources, including a tutorial on how to build measurable objectives. teachonline.asu.edu/objectives-builder
- Businessballs (2017). This resource provides Bloom's taxonomy with application tool kits. www.businessballs.com/self-awareness/blooms-taxonomy-6
- Educational Technology and Mobile Learning (2017). This resource publishes the Modern Taxonomy Wheel. www.educatorstechnology.com/2013/04/the-modern-taxonomy-wheel.html
- Wayne State University (2017). This resource helps you learn how to write SMART objectives. hr.wayne.edu/leads/phase1/smart-objectives

REFERENCES

Anderson, L. W., & Krathwohl, D. R. (2001). *A taxonomy for learning, teaching, and assessing.* New York, NY: Addison Wesley Longman.

Bean, J. C. (2011). *Engaging ideas: The professor's guide to integrating writing, critical thinking, and active learning in the classroom* (2nd ed.). San Francisco, CA: Jossey-Bass.

Bloom, B. (1956). *Taxonomy of educational objectives: The classification of educational goals.* New York, NY: Longmans, Green.

Fink, L. D. (2013). *Creating significant learning experiences: An integrated approach to designing college courses* (2nd ed.). San Francisco, CA: Jossey-Bass.

Keating, S. B. (2015). *Curriculum development and evaluation in nursing* (3rd ed.). New York, NY: Springer Publishing.

Kharbach, M. (2017). Educational technology and mobile learning. Retrieved from http://www .educatorstechnology.com/2013/04/the-modern-taxonomy-wheel.html

Knowles, M. S. (1984). *The adult learner: A neglected species.* Houston, TX: Gulf Publishing.

McKeachie, W., & Svinicki, M. (2014). *McKeachie's teaching tips: Strategies, research, and theories for college and university teachers* (14th ed.). Boston, MA: Houghton Mifflin.

Murray, H., Gillese, E., Lennon, M., Mercer, P., & Robinson, M. (1996). American Association of Higher Education bulletin. Retrieved from https://www.aahea.org/index.php/aahea-bulletin

National League for Nursing. (2013). Ethical principles for nursing education. Retrieved from http:// www.nln.org/docs/default-source/default-document-library/ethical-principles-for-nursing-education -final-final-010312.pdf?sfvrsn=2

Nilson, L. (2016). *Teaching at its best: A research-based resource for college instructors* (4th ed.). San Francisco, CA: Jossey-Bass.

Quality and Safety Education for Nurses Institute. (2017). QSEN competencies. Retrieved from http:// qsen.org/competencies

Raman, J. (2015). Mobile technology in nursing education: Where do we go from here? A review of the literature. *Nurse Education Today, 35,* 663–672. doi:10.1016/j.nedt.2015.01.018

S.M.A.R.T. Objectives. (2017). Wayne State University. Retreived from https://hr.wayne.edu/leads/ phase1/smart-objectives

Walvoord, B., Anderson, V., & Angelo, T. (2009). *Effective grading: A tool for learning and assessment* (2nd ed.). San Francisco, CA: Jossey-Bass.

Wiggins, G., & McTighe, J. (2006). *Understanding by design* (2nd ed.). Alexandria, VA: Association for Supervision & Curriculum Development.

Zimmerman, B., Plsek, P., & Lindberg, C. (2008). *Edgeware: Insights from complexity science for health care leaders* (3rd ed.). Irving, TX: Plexus Institute.

CHAPTER 5

Evidence-Based Practice: Gaining and Using the Evidence With Technology

CHAPTER GOAL

Gain an overview of information literacy and its competencies, which students need to access and appropriately implement the current science of learning that undergirds best practices.

BEGINNING REFLECTION

1. What does the concept of information literacy mean to you?
2. If you are currently teaching, how do you help your students search the literature? If you are not teaching, what is your approach for searching the literature?
3. How can your approach be updated to keep up with new access to information and technologies?
4. What are the legal and ethical implications of using new technologies, such as blogs, during the information literacy process?

Overheard: *How many articles do I have to put on my reference list?*

Clinical education is rapidly changing, and our students and graduates need tools to keep up. The web changes the amount of information we can access, as well as how we access that information. In the past, students likely prepared to care for patients by having one good textbook and hoping it covered the complexity of their patients. Now students can prepare, in essence, with a universe of knowledge that is open to them. The challenge is that they can become lost in that universe without some guidance. Now the textbook (digital or hardcopy) more likely serves as a basic guide, with additional websites required for further topic detail or ongoing updates.

Clinicians have deficiencies in how to search, evaluate, and apply the best evidence (Institute of Medicine [IOM], 2003). Information literacy and evidence-based practice (EBP) are two key concepts that can help bridge an education and practice gap. Varied nursing organizations recognize these as essential. For example:

- The *Essentials of Baccalaureate Education for Professional Nursing Practice* identifies computer skills and information literacy as competencies required by undergraduate nursing programs (American Association of Colleges of Nursing, 2008).
- The American Nurses Association (2014) has described information literacy as a critical concept in supporting EBP.

Information literacy concepts are also consistent with lifelong learning, which will be essential to all healthcare professionals and educators. The purpose of this chapter is to discuss information literacy as a central concept in teaching with technologies. The chapter describes steps to help faculty, students, and clinicians use technology as a process for accessing information resources. Strategies for helping students access, critique, and use resources in meaningful ways are chapter themes.

INFORMATION LITERACY: WHAT DOES IT MEAN?

Information literacy serves as a tool and foundation for lifelong learning and a basis for further work with technologies. Information literacy consists of cognitive skills, technical skills, and knowledge. In 2013, the Association of College & Research Libraries (ACRL) Board of Directors approved the Information Literacy Competency Standards for Nursing (ILCSN), which states that information-literate nurses (students and clinicians) should be able to:

1. Identify the type and amount of information needed.
2. Access appropriate information in an effective and efficient manner.
3. Critique the acquired information and modify the search, if necessary.
4. Use the information to achieve their goal(s).
5. Implement the entire process in a legal and ethical manner.

Why do some students find it so confusing to search the literature and/or use what is found there? Rapid advances in technologies such as the Internet have led to almost unlimited access to information. Although it is fairly easy to access vast amounts of information, it is more challenging to ensure that students understand the worth of that information and interpret it correctly. Data suggest that students experience the following challenges with information literacy (Appel, 2006):

- Identifying trustworthy and useful information
- Managing excessive information
- Effectively communicating information

With volumes of information available, the concepts and processes for attaining information literacy will be valuable for students' work in the future. Faculty have an opportunity to provide direction in learning this important skill.

RELATED CONCEPTS

Information literacy and EBP are overlapping concepts. Accessing and using literature efficiently provide an evidence base for clinical practice. In terms of helping students work with patients, information literacy is consistent with EBP. Additional related terms include *reading literacy* and *health literacy*. These sound similar but are different concepts. All of these terms are important in helping students and their future patients understand health information. Computer literacy is also considered a component of information literacy. Descriptors of selected terms for discussion purposes include the following:

- *Information literacy* relates to skills or competencies needed to efficiently maneuver through the vast amounts of information available.
- *EBP*, in simple terms, means basing clinical practice on the best evidence available. The goal is to use evidence from a well-developed body of research. When research is missing, best evidence has been extended to include best practices coming from theory and expert clinicians.
- *Research utilization* might be considered an extension of EBP to include a focus on using well-developed research as a basis for clinical decisions.
- *Computer literacy* involves knowing how to use and manage the computer skills required in information literacy.
- *Reading literacy* relates to general reading ability.
- *Health literacy* is the ability to read and understand with a specific focus on health-related issues (IOM, 2004).

HOW DO WE HELP STUDENTS LEARN INFORMATION LITERACY?

General Principles

Help students understand why they must conduct literature reviews. An important first step is helping students understand why they are being asked to review the literature. Beginning students have often become accustomed to faculty or the textbook gathering and synthesizing the information they need to know. With literature searches, we ask students to transition from readers of texts to those who find, critique, and synthesize diverse resources. Fewer skills are needed to review a text that has all the information synthesized in one place than to find, critique, and synthesize information from a variety of web-based resources.

Update search methods to reflect available technologies. The concept of searching the literature has changed with the advent of the web. When it comes to technology and information literacy, we ask students and future practitioners to take on new roles. We used to have students read a textbook or, in more advanced contexts, spend hours in the library with some version of a large cumulative index from which sources were identified, reviewed, and documented on bibliography cards. With the wealth of information now online, that system has limited use and students are better served if we update the methods for teaching literature searches to reflect the new realities of technology. The Internet is now the easiest and fastest source of current literature, and that reality must be reflected in the information literacy processes that we teach.

Fingertip technology is a term used to describe easy access to clinical information. Mobile computing devices such as smartphones and notebook computers can be used in systematic searches and retrieval of evidence-based protocols at point of care. The main advantages to fingertip technologies are portability and clinical point-of-care access. Particularly for students who are still learning the basics, these tools provide an important way to rapidly access information for changing patient needs. Many interest groups, including hospitals, specialty groups, and governmental agencies, are intent on exploring how technologies can promote information literacy and a strong evidence base to enhance the quality of patient care. These devices can also assist clinicians in providing quality care through point-of-care clinical documentation.

Teach basic strategies for beginners and more advanced strategies for advanced students. The novice-to-expert model (Benner, 2001) supports transitions in gaining skills for information literacy and EBP. These competencies relate to a skill set for EBP, with competencies designed specifically for varied program levels from undergraduate to doctoral. This is true within program levels as well, in which students earlier in a program learn more basic content, which is foundational to content taught to students further along in the program (Dotson et al., 2015).

Recognizing Professional Literature

Faculty may need to teach beginners how to recognize professional literature. An amazing variety of data sources are available online, and the boundaries between professional and other types of data are often blurred. Further issues arise because print sources can often be accessed online. It is important that teachers help students recognize what is and is not professional literature. For beginning students, this may be as basic as creating criteria by assignment type or stipulating that professional references should include an identifiable author, publication source, and date of publication. More advanced students, for example, may be further directed to only use peer-reviewed sources.

Being Systematic in Finding and Accessing Information

Because so much data are accessible, faculty need to help students understand how to begin and refine literature searches. Technology makes it easy to access resources for guiding clinical practice, but finding the best resources can be challenging. Faculty can help students understand the basics of systematic review as a key component of information literacy. Use of electronic resources leads to the potential for promoting more efficient use of best evidence.

The current mass of available information makes it impossible to review all of the literature. No longer can one claim that all of the literature was reviewed, as invariably some part of the literature was missed. Instead, we strive for a well-documented systematic review, but today's worldwide library also makes it less clear what a thorough search entails. It is no wonder the changing concept of *search* may be confusing for students.

A systematic search refers to a search strategy that is so well described that it can be reproduced. Faculty can guide students, particularly more advanced students, in the following ways:

- Describe what is meant by the term *systematic search* and why it is important.
- Frame the search. Framing includes describing concepts and terms used in the search as well as the database searched. This also includes clarifying terms—that is, taking terms from a fuzzy concept to something recognizable in the literature.
- Identify key words to search. Describing concepts is a project in and of itself and requires ongoing attention. Students may start by looking up words they think represent their concept of interest, and then they may advance to searching for word combinations. Another helpful approach is to review the standard search terms within a variety of search engines. Once relevant search terms are identified, conduct a brief search to determine whether the articles produced match the concept you are trying to find.
- Think about the questions you want to ask the literature. Understand that the data you find are determined by the questions you ask. For example, asking how to teach diabetic patients about their medicine yields different information than asking how to teach diabetic patients to give themselves an insulin shot.
- Be thoughtful about databases. Most students currently have access to a variety of databases and search options. Which databases are best for answering questions? Again, the answer depends on the questions asked. Guide students in searching outside common professional databases as necessitated by the problem identified. Many traditional databases are still relevant today, as represented in Exhibit 5.1. In addition, the Internet has spawned a wide variety of other search engines, such as Google Scholar Search, Yahoo! Search, and the Internet Archive Search, which may initially be more familiar to the general population of students as they start their professional education.
- Discuss what counts as an acceptable literature/evidence source at the outset. This includes if and how diverse websites or other resources such as blogs or wikis fit. For example, will an assignment be directed toward students gaining professional references from traditional literature or will other resources be accepted?
- Partner with faculty/librarians for searches. Faculty/librarian teams are beneficial for developing assignments, framing searches, and tracking elusive publications. Even a technology expert can benefit from the

EXHIBIT 5.1

SAMPLE HEALTH PROFESSIONS DATABASES AND ELECTRONIC RESOURCES

CUMULATIVE INDEX TO NURSING AND ALLIED HEALTH LITERATURE (CINAHL)

What It Is: broad selection of nursing and allied health citations
Key Features: links to full text if available and email alerts available

ACCESSMEDICINE

What It Is: online collection of medical reference books and tools
Key Features: includes drug guides, images, patient care, decision-making tools, and patient education

COCHRANE LIBRARY

What It Is: a collection of databases designed to provide evidence for decision making
Key Features: provides an excellent resource for systematic reviews

PROQUEST NURSING & ALLIED HEALTH DATABASE

What It Is: database of nursing and allied health citations
Key Features: includes The Joanna Briggs Institute evidence-based best-practice information sheets, systematic reviews, and evidence summaries

PUBMED

What It Is: searchable medical literature database covering selected international biomedical journals that provide clinical and biomedical literature citations
Key Features: includes links to online full-text, clinical queries, and email alerts available

MEDLINEPLUS

What It Is: searchable full-text consumer-level health information database
Key Features: encyclopedia, dictionaries, images, clinical trial information, and tutorials

TRIP (TURNING RESEARCH INTO PRACTICE)

What It Is: searches of numerous evidence-based resources
Key Features: offers evidence-based medicine, images, and searches patient information pamphlets

Adapted with permission from Whitehair, C. (2009). *Sample health professions databases and electronic resources.* Unpublished manuscript, University of Kansas Medical Center, Kansas City, Kansas.

expertise of a good librarian who has gained exquisite search skills on a variety of topics. Changing one simple nuance can make the difference between finding little to no relevant information to opening a barrage of previously unrealized sources.

Thinking Critically and Critiquing

Many online resources are available to students, and many of these have been developed without professional peer review. This discussion has focused primarily on professional print publications for critique, but as students seek online resources to review, options among these resources can become quite complex. Faculty need to first guide students in differentiating between a range of online resources, varying from professional journal databases and websites to very basic lay information (with many shades between), and then assist students with guidelines for critical evaluation of these diverse web resources.

Some of the different kinds of material students may access are reliable and valid, and some are not. Although professional references such as journal articles already use criteria for literature critique, the reliability and validity of other types of resources, such as lay and professional websites, must be critiqued. Students have access to lots of information and may need help determining which sources are legitimate and which are not, and resources for teaching this are becoming available. Five criteria (accuracy, authority, objectivity, currency, and coverage) are recommended for review of web pages by CCCOnline Library (2017). The University of Wisconsin–Green Bay (UWGB, 2017) suggests evaluating the web page author, date, sources, domain, site design, and writing style.

This same review process applies to the myriad online resources that exist in other formats (e.g., videos and podcasts) and for various uses (e.g., patient education resources, drug guides). Expanded guidelines for critiquing online videos are now emerging. Instructors should stress to students the importance of determining whether these resources are quality products or simply commercials. Students need to gain critique strategies for the varied resources now available online. Approaches to information search and critique must keep changing as new sources of information emerge.

Once information from an acceptable source is found, the process for teaching further critique varies, depending on the students' level of education. One basic consideration for all students is their ability to describe the level of evidence presented in a particular resource. For example, all students should understand that quantitative studies are at a higher end of the continuum, followed by qualitative studies, institutional databases, and clinical expertise (IOM, 2003). A variety of resources exist for teaching critique strategies and helping students at all levels to access the best evidence online. Exhibit 5.2

EXHIBIT 5.2

REVIEW CRITERIA FOR HEALTH INFORMATION ONLINE

The following provide guides to help students (and their patients) critique online resources related to health care:

- *A User's Guide to Finding and Evaluating Health Information on the Web: Medical Library Association*: www.mlanet.org/resources/userguide.html
- *Evaluating Internet Health Information: A Tutorial from the National Library of Medicine*: www.nlm.nih.gov/medlineplus/webeval/webeval.html

provides additional resources to assist students with their online review of health information.

Synthesizing and Communicating

Synthesizing means combining the information found and making sense of the literature recommendations. It requires reflection and critical thinking and includes looking for strengths and weaknesses, similarities and differences, and/or gaps in the literature evidence. This critical reflection guides students in making summary statements about the evidence derived from the various sources. Did the literature reflect only qualitative studies by three authors, or were there multiple randomized controlled studies by 10 different researchers? Were there no research studies at all, but only blog discussions about a topic? Did your search yield findings on the cardiac patient population you were searching for, but not in the home care context that you were seeking? Given the findings summary, what are the implications for your own work?

INFORMATION LITERACY AND EBP

How does EBP relate to information literacy and clinical practice applications? The goal of EBP is to gain and use best evidence in helping patients and providers make choices in clinical care to promote safety, quality, and healthcare value (IOM, 2003). In teaching students' information literacy and EBP, we:

- Assess their current expertise or educational level.
- Orient them to both what they will be doing and why it is important.
- Engage them with relevant assignments that challenge (but do not overwhelm).
- Provide feedback based on the student level.

Faculty can direct students to use evidence-based resources in developing their assignments, even with something as basic as guidance in developing a health fair poster. For example, as students seek references to support their poster, faculty help them identify the differences between a self-help page on the web developed by one individual and the EBP resources from the National Institutes of Health or other national organizations. In asking students to use the best science (or evidence) in their projects, faculty might direct beginning students developing a depression awareness poster to use an appropriate evidence base such as the National Institutes of Health or the Centers for Disease Control and Prevention.

As students advance with more complex assignments directed toward gaining an evidence base, critical thinking is enhanced as they consider the relevance of information they have searched and retrieved or syntheses they have found on a given topic. The focus now becomes the clinical problem and the population and context.

As we teach with technology, we are trying to help students develop self-directed learning habits for lifelong learning. This is particularly important when related to gaining tools for information literacy and EBP. Students, for example, find available online pamphlets they can provide to patients, but to be credible, the pamphlets need to be based on the best evidence. A faculty role includes helping students use best evidence in clinical decision making for needed practice changes. Initially faculty can help students to:

- Understand the need to identify and frame the clinical problem. This can be as basic as how to frame a clinical question to obtain the best literature search or evidence base. The mnemonic PICO (patient, intervention, comparison, and outcome) can be taught, for example, to help frame clinical questions (Melnyk & Fineout-Overholt, 2015).
- Begin clinical topic searches seeking systematic reviews, recalling the benefits of a well-done systematic review on a given topic.
- Evaluate evidence-based protocols for appropriateness with specific specialty populations.

The same evidence-based protocol may not be useful in all settings or for all patients. Although information literacy is about locating and evaluating information, EBP supports clinical decisions in the context in which they are applied. After gaining the best evidence on a topic, students need to learn to put the evidence gained into context, applying information appropriately to a given patient population and setting. Fall prevention is one example. Although basic fall-prevention concepts are relevant across settings, specific fall prevention protocols depend not only on physical environments, but also on patient characteristics. For example, for a patient with Parkinson's disease, the protocols would differ depending on the stage of the disease and the patient setting (e.g., home, hospital).

CREATING ALLIANCES

Beginning students may work with a good librarian, but more advanced students may also create partnerships or alliances with librarians and a wide variety of other health professionals. This approach can be a mutually beneficial way to combine and enhance knowledge and expertise. Benefits to these partnerships include the following:

- Communicating and collaborating. Teaming up with librarians reminds us what services are available and provides a good start to systematic reviews. The ACRS's (2016) Framework for Information Literacy for Higher Education provides key concepts with a variety of options for implementation.
- Reviewing evidence developed by other disciplines. We have opportunities for multiple disciplines to share and learn from one another's professional literature, helping students best understand the state of the

science on a topic area. Real benefit exists in adding a frame or perspective from another discipline in viewing and enhancing our evidence base for practice.

LEGAL AND ETHICAL IMPLICATIONS

Along with the many potential benefits of using technology to increase information literacy comes many potential risks, which increases the professional liability and responsibility of students and clinicians. Some concerns have not changed from pretechnology times. For example, when citing a reference found through a literature search, proper credit to the author must be cited and cited in an acceptable format and the detail of the citation increases when the author's exact words are used.

The everyday use of technology that now exists in almost all aspects of life exponentially increases the realm of additional concerns. This is especially true because of technology's ubiquitous and commonplace nature and our oftentimes mindless use of it. Today's students are used to sharing their daily activities on Facebook or Snapchat, and little attention is likely paid to posts about their workday. It might be easy to think that someone will see the post and help the student figure out what to do for the 72-year-old patient with cardiac disease in room 2389, without consciously realizing the violation of confidentiality. The National Council of State Boards of Nursing (2011) has issued a white paper guiding the use of social media in nursing. The paper takes a broad approach that applies to many uses of technology, including information literacy. Particularly concerned with protecting patients' choices to disclose personal information (privacy) and the way that shared information is subsequently handled by healthcare providers (confidentiality), the National Council reviews problems associated with social and electronic media, as well as possible consequences of its misuse.

Although a literature search through a professional search engine may be fairly straightforward, searching a blog for information may lead an unwitting student to divulge personal information about the patient in a public venue. Despite being careful to avoid the patient's name, even providing age, diagnosis, and room number (as mentioned previously) makes the patient identifiable, since many Facebook friends likely know where you work. Instructors should warn students and clinicians that (a) no information that can identify a patient or student can be shared without a specific need to know, (b) posts are not private and reach far beyond the intended recipient, (c) deleted items do not really disappear entirely, (d) it is never appropriate to make derogatory comments about anyone online, and (e) personal devices should not be used in one's professional role. Be sure to know and follow your employer's policies and procedures regarding the use of both the institution's and your own personal technological devices for work-related matters. Also, violating these legal and ethical principles can lead to board of nursing actions, loss of employment, and even civil or criminal penalties.

SUMMARY

As clinicians emerge from our educational programs, it is important that they have skills for information literacy and know the process for EBP to serve as good clinicians for their patients. In the health professions education report (IOM, 2003), a quality gap is described as the care that patients receive versus the care that patients should receive. Information literacy and EBP, based on informed clinicians knowing how to access the best-practice knowledge, is one contribution to narrowing that quality gap. Once we help students understand the basics, such as what counts as professional literature, our focus will be to help them think critically about both the process for searching and the criteria for critique. Faculty provide leadership that helps students understand what professional literature is, find the best clinical evidence, critique it, and apply the information in appropriate contexts, all while following established legal and ethical guidelines.

ENDING REFLECTIONS FOR YOUR LEARNING NOTEBOOK

1. What is the most important content that you learned in this chapter?
2. What are your plans for using the information provided in this chapter in your future teaching endeavors?
3. What are your further learning goals?

GUIDELINES FOR TEACHING AND LEARNING WITH TECHNOLOGIES

Quick Teaching Tips

1. Involve librarian partners in working with students to enhance their search skills and broaden their information literacy.
2. Create assignments that help students identify the ways that an evidence base is currently used in their clinical setting (e.g., reviewing protocols or clinical pathways on a topic).

Questions for Further Reflection

1. Where does information literacy belong in the curriculum?
2. What are the similarities and differences in learning needs related to EBP for beginning health professions students and advanced graduate students?
3. How do we integrate the concept of EBP across a curriculum so that all faculty have the same goal? Are there best practices to guide us in this endeavor?

Learning Activity: Systematic Review and Search for the Best Evidence Survey

The purpose of this activity is to further students' reflection on, and interaction with, chapter content. The prompts can be used as a beginning self-assessment of knowledge about systematic review, or they could serve as a class discussion guide.

Answer Agree or Disagree to each of the following statements related to literature review seeking best evidence on a topic.[1]

1. ____A practical screen and methodological screen for including excluding articles in literature reviews are the same thing.
2. ____An online literature search is typically a sufficient approach to the review of the literature.
3. ____Searching one database should cover most educational research topics.
4. ____Finding the key words in an article title makes this a good match for your literature review.
5. ____Descriptive reviews rely on reviewer experiences and evidence, whereas a meta-analysis uses statistical techniques to combine study results.
6. ____A written list of decisions made relates primarily to your research method section.
7. ____A literature review is systematic, explicit, and reproducible.
8. ____Inclusion and exclusion criteria are important concepts for a literature review.
9. ____A screening protocol can promote consistency and quality in a review.
10. ____Descriptive reviews identify and interpret similarities and differences in literature purpose, methods, and findings.
11. ____A standardized review protocol can be helpful in clarifying inclusion/exclusion criteria.
12. ____When completing a literature review, once your search criteria are set, no changes should be made.
13. ____Once a research literature review is completed, a synthesis report should be generated to summarize and identify themes and gaps in the literature.
14. ____In completing literature reviews, it can be useful to develop a matrix that allows one to organize results by topics such as type of article and year of publication.
15. ____After completing a descriptive literature review to answer specific questions, the reviewer has a responsibility to disseminate and make the information as accessible as possible.

Survey concepts developed from Garrard, J. (2006). *Health sciences literature review made easy: The matrix method* (2nd ed.). Boston, MA: Jones & Bartlett.

[1] Responses 1, 2, 3, 4, 6, and 12 are considered "Disagree"; all others are considered "Agree."

Online Resources for Further Learning

■ American Library Association. This association provides a variety of resources on information literacy and tips for working with students. www.ala.org

■ Academic Center for Evidence-Based Practice (ACE). This center provides diverse online resources for educators as well as ongoing workshops on teaching EBP. nursing.uthscsa.edu/onrs/starmodel/

REFERENCES

American Association of Colleges of Nursing. (2008). The essentials of baccalaureate education for professional nursing practice. Retrieved from http://www.aacnnursing.org/Portals/42/Publications/BaccEssentials08.pdf

American Nurses Association. (2014). *Nursing informatics: Practice scope and standards of practice* (2nd ed.). Silver Spring, MD: Author.

Appel, J. (2006). Report: Students struggle with information literacy. *eSchool News.* Retrieved from https://www.eschoolnews.com/2006/11/28/report-students-struggle-with-information-literacy

Association of College & Research Libraries. (2013). Information literacy competency standards for nursing. Retrieved from http://www.ala.org/acrl/standards/nursing

Association of College & Research Libraries. (2016). Framework for Information Literacy for Higher Education. Retrieved from http://www.ala.org/acrl/standards/ilframework

Benner, P. (2001). *From novice to expert: excellence and power in clinical nursing practice* (Commemorative ed.). Upper Saddle River, NJ: Prentice Hall.

CCCOnline Library. (2017). Learn about evaluating sources: Five criteria for evaluating web pages. Retrieved from https://ccconline.libguides.com/c.php?g=242130&p=1609638

Dotson, B. J., Lewis, L. S., Aucoin, J. W., Murray, S., Chapin, D., & Walters, P. (2015). Teaching evidence-based practice (EBP) across a four-semester nursing curriculum. Retrieved from http://www.jtln.org/article/S1557-3087(15)00040-2/fulltext

Garrard, J. (2006). *Health sciences literature review made easy: The matrix method* (2nd ed.). Boston, MA: Jones & Bartlett.

Institute of Medicine. (2003). *Health professions education: A bridge to quality.* Washington, DC: National Academies Press.

Institute of Medicine. (2004). Health literacy: A prescription to end confusion. Retrieved from http://www.nationalacademies.org/hmd/Reports/2004/Health-Literacy-A-Prescription-to-End-Confusion.aspx

Melnyk, B. M., & Fineout-Overholt, E. (2015). *Evidence-based practice in nursing & healthcare: A guide to best practice* (3rd ed.). Philadelphia, PA: Wolters Kluwer.

National Council of State Boards of Nursing. (2011). White paper: A nurse's guide to the use of social media. Retrieved from https://www.ncsbn.org/3874.htm

University of Wisconsin–Green Bay. (2017). Computing & information technology: How can I tell if a website is credible? Retrieved from https://uknowit.uwgb.edu/page.php?id=30276

Whitehair, C. (2009). *Sample health professions databases and electronic resources.* Unpublished manuscript, University of Kansas Medical Center, Kansas City, Kansas.

Faculty as Learning Facilitators With Technology

Creating Learning Teams: Basics for Safe/Effective Communication

CHAPTER GOAL

Consider good communication practices to guide teaching with technologies and facilitate civil, respectful communication in a variety of situations.

BEGINNING REFLECTION

1. How does technology affect your current communications?
2. What are your current communication approaches when teaching with technologies for different purposes and for different audiences, such as individuals versus groups?
3. How do different communication techniques facilitate civil and respectful interactions?
4. How can interprofessional education be fostered with tech-savvy communication?
5. What role does good communication play in the provision of safe, quality patient care?

Overheard: *Do students really think it is okay to send demanding emails to faculty?*

Communication is the cornerstone of our relationships with others. Be it verbal, nonverbal, handwritten, text-based, in person, or virtual, communication provides the means by which people relate to one another and convey their thoughts, feelings, and ideas to others. Communication ranges from the most personal and intimate communication to the most impersonal and indifferent.

In today's world, it often feels that there is no escape from the constant barrage of incoming messages. Technology makes it possible to reach anyone, anywhere, anytime. There are more and more communication options available to us, from cell phones and text messages to communication within learning management systems. How do we keep up with all the possible means of communication? How do we manage the influx of messages and respond appropriately in content, manner, and time? Given the 24/7 nature of today's communication, how do we somehow manage the sheer number of messages needing a response? Which ones take priority?

On a very different but equally important note, how can technology be used to communicate effectively with our students and healthcare communities? Because of the muting of facial expressions, gestures, and vocal inflections across video or computer screens, or their absence in the case of text-based communication, the effectiveness of communication can be limited. This stripping away of nonverbal communication can make meaning more difficult to interpret. Differing opinions, values, perspectives, cultures, and languages oftentimes complicate communication further. Add to this complexity the potential life-and-death nature of healthcare-related conversations, and the importance of good communication for nurses becomes apparent.

WHY IS COMMUNICATION IMPORTANT IN TEACHING TECHNOLOGIES?

Communication is important as the cornerstone of relationships with students and peers, as a tool to facilitate learning and critical thinking skills, and as a mechanism by which to improve the safety and quality of patient care. Communication "focuses on how people use messages to generate meaning within and across all kinds of contexts, cultures, channels and media" (National Communication Association, 2009). Communication is a learned process that consists of verbal, nonverbal, and electronic messages. Healthcare communication is often complicated by the life-and-death, hierarchical, and legal aspects of healthcare itself. Today those complexities have increased with the explosion of technologies that offer to facilitate, but can just as easily derail, communication efforts. Faculty are called on to be good communicators in a variety of situations, with a variety of individuals or groups, using a variety of technologies. The importance of communication is illustrated by its impact on relationships, civility, learning and critical thinking, safe and quality patient care, and health literacy.

Relationships

Effective communication is an essential element in the teacher–student relationship. Faculty must be able to communicate clear expectations to individual students, as well as to groups of students. Of course, students have a responsibility to express confusion and ask questions when faculty expectations and direction are not clear but, again, the faculty must then respond with clear direction. The onus is on faculty to communicate clearly, concisely, and appropriately, all in a timely manner.

It is also up to faculty to model professional communication to their students. The Quality and Safety Education for Nurses (QSEN) Institute (QSEN, 2017) project includes teamwork and collaboration as a competency in which nurses work effectively with, have open communication and respect for, and share decision making with other nurses and interprofessional teams to provide safe and quality care. Role modeling professional communication includes a broad range of skills, including collegial communication with peers, interdisciplinary communication within healthcare teams, and direct communication with patients and/or students.

Civility in Teaching and Learning

The goal of the teaching and learning environment is to create a place (physical or virtual) that fosters a community of leaners engaged in respectful inter-actions with the goal of enhancing their individual, as well as collective, edu-cation. Incivility, defined as disruptive and rude behavior, directly inhibits this respectful culture of learning and is on the increase in education. Clark and Springer (2010) conducted a study of both students' and faculty's uncivil behaviors. A student's uncivil behaviors included technology-oriented actions such as cell phone use, texting, and computer misuse in the classroom, as well as rude comments, side conversations, sleeping, and coming and going at times other than the official class schedule. Other student actions included bully-ing, cheating, having a sense of entitlement, blaming others, and marginalizing other students. Faculty displayed uncivil behavior toward students, such as demeaning behaviors, unreasonable demands, and not appreciating student contributions, as well as uncivil behaviors toward faculty peers and administra-tors. Literally, all behaviors identified as uncivil relate to communication, be they verbal, nonverbal, text-based, or some other form. Clark (2017) suggests that content on civility, along with closely related topics of professionalism and ethics, be implemented as early as new student orientation and subsequently integrated across the entire curriculum.

Learning and Critical Thinking

Communication has traditionally been used to evaluate how much learning has taken place. Students have been asked to communicate, via paper and pencil tests, online examinations, and formal papers, the extent to which they have mastered required content. What is often less recognized is the importance of communication to the learning process itself. For example, writing activities can be used not only to evaluate learning, but also to facilitate the learning process. Online, text-based discussions are examples of written assignments that can be used to teach critical thinking skills.

Safe, Quality Patient Care

Good communication skills are essential to safe, quality patient care. Perhaps this truth is best recognized in its absence. "Communication failure, a leading source of adverse events in healthcare, was involved in approximately 75% of more than 7,000 root cause analysis reports to the Department of Veterans Affairs National Center for Patient Safety" (Dunn et al., 2007, p. 317). Although this study was not updated, ongoing concerns exist. This statistic highlights the fact that teaching students improved communication skills is essential and can directly improve the quality of healthcare.

Health Literacy

The concept of health literacy is central to safe patient care, especially when communicating with and teaching diverse patients. Concepts of healthcare literacy are central to patient education, with cultural diversity, health literacy, and patient teaching being intertwined topics. As noted, communication failures are considered a major problem in current healthcare systems. Teaching health literacy skills is particularly important because once students have become comfortable with healthcare vocabulary, they may not remember that these terms are often confusing to patients. Students have limited impact on patients, healthcare systems, and public health unless they focus on effective communication skills and health literacy. Sample resources for helping students gain skills in health literacy are provided in Exhibit 6.1.

TEXT-BASED, COMPUTER-MEDIATED COMMUNICATION

Computer-mediated communication has become a major factor in our world, and as often happens as things evolve, semantics can be problematic. Many text-based communications are computer-mediated, but that is not always true (i.e., this book is text-based but not computer-mediated). Conversely, many computer-mediated communications are text-based but, again, that is not always true (i.e., podcasts and Skype). Our focus here is on communication that is both text-based and computer-mediated.

EXHIBIT 6.1

HEALTH LITERACY RESOURCES FOR FURTHER LEARNING

- *Health Literacy.* Resources are provided by the Health Resources and Services Administration, including free programs for online training: www.hrsa.gov/about/organization/bureaus/ohe/health-literacy/index.html
- *Health Literacy, a Prescription to End Confusion.* An online text from the IOM provides a variety of readings to guide students in learning to improve their work in health literacy www.nap.edu/catalog/10883/health-literacy-a-prescription-to-end-confusion

IOM, Institute of Medicine.

Text-based, computer-mediated communication can be either synchronous or asynchronous. *Synchronous* means that the people in communication with one another are communicating at the same time, whereas *asynchronous* means that the parties are not required to communicate with one another at the same time. These terms have been used extensively in online education but can also have relevance in other venues. Public and private communications are additional categories to consider. We can focus on communication to an individual or convey messages to groups, large or small. Eduscapes (2008a) provides further comments specific to online communication.

As text-based, computer-mediated communication replaces verbal communication, the expectations and uses of writing itself are changing. Most verbal communication was once casual, and written communication was often more formal. Now, although formal writing (such as scholarly papers) still exists, much written communication is more informal, and the standards for traditional, formal writing do not fit this new informal written communication style. For example, proper nouns and names are frequently not capitalized, and slang acronyms (such as "LOL," for "laughing out loud") abound. The transition from traditional, formal writing styles to contemporary, more informal writing styles presents a challenge for faculty, as students come with a focus on text-based lingo and faculty try to determine what is acceptable professionally.

Fortunately, a growing number of practice guides for the differing technological options are available. A good, broadly based communication guide that applies across all situations, including the Internet, is found in Shea's (1994) classic book, *Netiquette*, in which she identifies 10 core rules that still serve well in most cases. These rules, like theoretical foundations and best practices, remain fairly constant regardless of the specific text-based communication used. For example, Shea reminds us that, even in cyberspace, there are human beings at the other end of our communication, and those people deserve to have their time and privacy respected. Equally important is to use the same standards of behavior online that you would use in person. These fundamental concepts remain relevant today, although the boundaries between personal and professional communication are becoming more blurred (Engard, 2016). The seven must-know netiquette rules for professional behavior (Polished, 2017) include a reminder that your cyber fingerprint is always traceable and warnings to avoid posting unprofessional pictures, profanity, and/or divulging employer secrets.

GUIDES FOR COMMUNICATING WITH STUDENTS

Although the explosion of technology provides an opportunity to use any of the large variety of technological options for any given communication, the general principles of good communication apply regardless of the form of communication used (even old-fashioned, face-to-face communication). New technologies do mean, however, that faculty are in the position of having many choices and they need to make informed, responsible decisions about which technologies to use. Sometimes the simplest of those decisions are the hardest. For example, how does one handle the multiple messages (be they phone or text-based messages) that arrive daily from students? Basic tips include the following:

1. Make informed and responsible decisions on the mechanism by which you respond to the students. Just because a student e-mailed you does not mean you need to respond via e-mail. Sometimes a quick phone call is the best way to clarify complicated questions or situations.
2. Clarify to whom you should respond. If you are responding to a student with information that everyone in a course needs to know, then use a communication technique capable of including the entire class in the response. If you are responding to a student with personal or negative information, respond only to the individual directly.
3. Respond at a set time each day, limit that time, and tell students what your communication schedule is. One strategy used to manage the constant barrage of e-mails is to ignore the temptation to read and respond to them all day long. If you answer e-mail once a day at noon, tell students so that they know what to expect; if you plan to avoid or limit weekend responses, let students know that is your practice.
4. Give extra thought to the delivery of bad news (such as negative feedback on a paper or a poor grade). Blunt comments via text-based communication can come across as scathing, so take precautions to soften the message or use a face-to-face (or some other form of verbal communication) method that provides more input than simply the words used.
5. Pick the mode of your communication to fit the situation. Verbal communication provides noted benefits, but if you want a written record of sending the message and its receipt, e-mail can be a good option. Conversely, if you do not need a paper trail of the communication, or risk its being sent to someone else, then do not write it down.

ADDITIONAL CONSIDERATIONS ABOUT COMMUNICATION IN TEACHING AND LEARNING

Almost everything we do in education is communication based. Therefore, the importance of communication (and advances in technology to enhance communication) affects most everything, including writing assignments, class discussions, feedback and evaluation, social learning spaces, special communication needs, and interprofessional education (IPE).

Writing Assignments

Writing is one of the best critical thinking activities; hence the concept of writing to learn has become commonplace. Traditionally we have thought of writing as a mechanism to demonstrate and evaluate the completion of the learning process, such as end-of-semester term papers. These final products are considered high-stakes writing because they are usually graded only one time for accuracy, completeness, and scholarly format. An example is the term paper that is due toward the end of a course and that often represents a large portion of the course grade. An alternate approach is to require the same term paper assignment but design it to be completed in parts throughout the semester. Breaking the paper down into smaller assignments provides an opportunity for students to gain feedback along the way and learn by improving the assignment before submitting the entire paper at the semester's end. This step-by-step approach would be considered a lower-stakes form of writing evaluation.

Writing to learn also refers to the use of writing as a key component of the learning process. The purpose is not to document completed learning, but to facilitate the learning process itself, such as through journaling. In this case, the purpose of writing is to stimulate thoughts and connections between content and to engage students with the content to be learned. Such writing is usually informal, messy, and not edited to perfection. It is not graded per se, although credit may be given for its completion. This low-stakes writing offers many benefits, such as identifying misunderstandings, improving discussion, providing practice in writing, providing individualized insight into each student, and improving more formal writing projects.

Class Discussions

Basic principles of discussions hold true regardless of whether a technological format is used or if discussions are face to face in classrooms. Discussions across settings have the same issues, such as how prepared students are (or are not) for the discussion and how much the instructor should (or should not) participate. Although discussions have long been used as learning tools, online discussions have forced faculty to become more conscious and explicit in communicating guidelines to students. Some tips to direct discussions (whether classroom or online) include the following:

1. Determine the purpose of the discussion and how best it should be orchestrated. Using objectives, such as with a lesson plan format, provides direction for gaining desired outcomes.
2. Orient students to course discussion guidelines, including the expected frequency of student participation and the extent of participation recommended.
3. Clearly define your role as faculty in the discussion and communicate that to students. Too much faculty participation can smother a discussion, but too little can result in misinformation or wandering off topic. Particularly in online discussions, let students know when they can expect to hear from faculty.
4. If the class is large, breaking it up into smaller groups can be helpful. Optimal group size can vary, depending on the nature of the discussion,

but group size should be compatible with the discussion purpose and type and the amount of participation recommended.

5. Provide clear, concise evaluation criteria so that, if students will be graded on a discussion, they know the criteria. Faculty decisions about criteria include all aspects of participation that is evaluated, such as the frequency and quality of response. A simple rubric can outline faculty expectations.

6. Use interesting prompts and pose focused, open-ended questions to begin discussions and keep the discussions going. Sample prompts are provided by Eduscapes (2008b).

Feedback and Evaluation

Keeping a focus on the desired learning outcome for the students, which is the overall goal of the communication, promotes feedback as a learning tool. Providing questions and prompts to promote communication with the student can facilitate the ongoing learning process.

Discussed in more detail in Chapter 9, feedback and evaluation are related (and sometimes overlapping) yet different processes. *Feedback* is the more general term in which comments and data about an action, behavior, or knowledge are designed to positively affect that action, behavior, or knowledge in the future. Feedback has been described as information communicated to students that is based on an assessment and that helps students reflect and work further with the information provided. This includes constructing self-knowledge relevant to course learning and setting further learning goals (Bonnel, Ludwig, & Smith, 2007). Evaluation is the systematic appraisal (of value, rightness, accuracy, and appropriateness) of an action, behavior, or knowledge.

Shea's (1994) rules of netiquette again remind us that, although many of today's communication techniques use impersonal gadgets, there is a person on the other end of our communications and we need to treat him or her with the requisite respect all humans deserve. The opportunity to soften bad news, through face-to-face or video mechanisms that afford more than just textual input, is important to keep in mind. At the very least, reading and rereading and editing the text-based message before sending it helps ensure that the message is softened as much as possible.

Social Learning Spaces

New communication opportunities can also lead to new challenges. Many faculty and students belong to social spaces such as Facebook. The increased interest in social networking may blur professional and personal boundaries. The question becomes whether it is appropriate for faculty to have access to students' personal profiles and, conversely, if students should have access to faculty members' personal profiles. The open, public nature of these sites and the enduring nature of written words could create potential problems if communication does not meet high professional standards.

Guidelines of appropriate boundaries between students and faculty need to be developed and followed. Attention needs to be paid to how or if a particular social space is relevant to educational uses. Faculty and students may have differing opinions on how to best use this type of technology in learning. If faculty decide to share pages with students, thoughtful consideration about what personal content is posted is recommended. Be careful, too, not to violate the Family Educational Rights and Privacy Act (FERPA) by disclosing any protected information about students. FERPA also protects the privacy of student educational records.

A related issue is faculty access to students' sites. Situations have been reported in which students have posted inappropriate information (e.g., examination questions and confidential information about patients) on their profiles. Such behavior becomes open to disciplinary action against these students. Whatever approach is taken, at the very least, the use of online social sites must be addressed in student orientations and through ongoing reminders.

In today's virtual world, learning spaces are understood to be any place where learning occurs. In this respect, social spaces offer one more opportunity for a learning space, and the challenge for educators is to make the best possible use of that space for the most appropriate learning experiences and content. Skiba, Connors, and Jeffries (2009) suggest the benefit of social networking tools created by faculty to support ongoing communities of practice, including students and professionals. Further discussion of learning communities is provided in Chapter 7.

Special Communication Needs

Faculty also need to remain cognizant of students with special needs. One such group might be students for whom English is a second (or new) language (ESL). Many ESL learners benefit from the nonverbal cues that visual communication and body language provide. Text-based communication, stripped of nonverbal cues to augment the words, is often more difficult for ESL students to interpret. Online technologies however do provide the opportunity to review archived discussions and to look up words in dictionaries. Evolving translator resources and online voice application technologies provide further opportunities for ESL students.

Technology-facilitated communication can be helpful to some students with special needs. The hearing impaired may benefit from text-based communication. Online courses may be particularly convenient for students with mobility impairments. Students with impaired digits, hands, or limbs may benefit from voice-activated technology that enables them to participate more fully in courses. Further study of best approaches is needed.

Interprofessional Education

The Interprofessional Education Collaborative (IPEC; 2016) identified four core IPE competencies: values/ethics, roles/responsibilities, interprofessional communication, and teams and teamwork. The core competency communication indicates that healthcare professionals should be responsive to patients, families, communities, and professionals; it can be used to both prevent disease and promote health. Communication has eight subcompetencies, such as appropriate use of communication tools and technologies, language that is understood by the persons/groups involved, active listening, timely and sensitive feedback, and the use of respectful language. The success of IPE has direct implications for the quality of care that patients receive in the healthcare system.

HEALTHCARE IMPLICATIONS

Good communication techniques are key not only in the classroom, but also for preparing students to work on clinical teams. Communication has a tremendous impact on the quality of healthcare. Institute of Medicine (IOM) reports (Finkelman & Kenner, 2014) have focused on quality care issues, paying particular attention to fragmented care and problems of communication within healthcare teams and between healthcare providers and patients, which have had a negative impact on quality healthcare. A 2009 report indicated that 75% of patients in a teaching hospital could not name the physician in charge of their inpatient care (Arora et al., 2009). Research over the past 30 years indicates that the provider's ability to communicate effectively has a strong impact on the patient's health outcomes, satisfaction, and overall care experience. For example, ineffective team communication is the cause of almost 66% of all medical errors between 1995 and 2005 (Institute for Healthcare Communication, 2011). Technology systems have been touted as a major approach for reducing communication errors. For example, computerized medical records and prescriber order-entry systems can promote safety by eliminating messy handwriting.

Computer-generated reminders can help reduce errors of omission. Online databases improve quality by ensuring that healthcare providers have access to the latest in evidence-based practice, and computerized decision-support systems can help standardize approaches. Electronic medical records can make data more complete by highlighting missing data and can make that information available instantaneously to other members of the healthcare team and to the patient. Communication itself can be facilitated using e-mail. Our students are prepared for clinical patient care only if they have comfort and skills with clinical technologies that enhance team communication.

As faculty, it is important to help students become familiar with the best communication practices for clinical agency work (and staff development) and the ways that technologies can help. Select considerations for discussion include the following:

■ Engage student and staff in ongoing work groups to guide further assessment and use of the best communication practices throughout a clinical agency. These ongoing discussion groups can extend education beyond awareness-raising to recommended applications.

- Make students and staff aware of the policies guiding the practice of patient-centered communication in a clinical agency. One topic includes respectful language using common terms (health literacy) that all would understand.
- Consider additional resources for when the patient does not use English as a first language. More information might be included in student and staff orientation about available resources and ways to access the policies and equipment.
- Promote open staff communication about potential concerns and near-miss communication problems by promoting a culture of quality and safety; an example could include debriefing after a situation when team function is not optimal.
- Add select resources to student and staff orientation such as "Speak-Up" (The Joint Commission, 2017) and "Ask Me 3" (Whaley, 2013) for use in engaging patients in their healthcare communication.
- Generate talking points to engage students and staff in further discussion related to specific clinical questions and concerns.

Civility in Healthcare

Just as incivility negatively impacts the teaching and learning environment, its presence in the healthcare context also affects the quality of healthcare itself and the healthcare environment in which we work. The Joint Commission (2008) claims that safe and quality patient care requires good communication and teamwork and cites uncivil behaviors as contributing to reduced patient satisfaction and increased adverse outcomes, cost of care, and staff vacancies. They recommend a lengthy list of actions to address this problem, including educating all team members, holding all team members accountable for modeling positive behaviors, enforcing consistent discipline that reinforces positive behavior and punishes negative actions, and developing policies and procedures that, among other things, provides for zero tolerance of uncivil behaviors.

Communication for Patient Safety in Healthcare

Summarizing findings from various sources, Gooch (2016) states that "communication failures were linked to 1,744 patient deaths in five years and $1.7 billion in malpractice costs" and that better communication among clinicians and patients could reduce hospital readmissions by 25%. Gooch claims that the problem of poor communication is difficult to address because (a) it is so pervasive that it impacts every aspect of healthcare; (b) communication itself is so complex because it is affected by past experience and relationships, upbringing, language skills, ethnicity, and personality; (c) changing communication skills is not amenable to a simple, intellectual approach; and (d) the hospital environment is chaotic by nature, which only complicates an already complicated matter. Interventions require the unwavering priority of putting the patient first. In addition to well-established suggestions, such as continual staff development, Gooch suggests the less traditional approach of medical improvisation in which experiential learning activities help teach and improve communication skills.

TeamSTEPPS® (Team Strategies and Tools to Enhance Performance and Patient Safety) is the response of the Agency for Healthcare Research and Quality's (AHRQ; 2016) to the problems with communication in healthcare. This evidence-based program is aimed at improving communication and teamwork among healthcare providers, with the aim of quality patient outcomes. Among their toolkit is a pocket guide that contains strategies for improving communication and behaviors that impact both safety and quality of patient care. Communication techniques include situation, background, assessment, and recommendation (SBAR); call-out; check-back; handoff; and introduction, patient, assessment, situation, safety—"the"—background, actions, timing, ownership, and next ("I PASS the BATON").

Health Literacy

Communication between the healthcare team and the patient and/or family is as important as the communication among the healthcare team. Health literacy is the extent to which patients/family can gain, process, and understand their health information and care options to make informed healthcare decisions (Office of Disease Prevention and Health Promotion [ODPHP], 2017a). Although there are certainly vulnerable populations in respect to health literacy (e.g., older adults, people with less than a high school education, and non-native English speakers), the National Assessment of Adult Literacy (NAAL; 2006) found that only 12% of all adults have proficient health literacy. Limited health literacy is associated with the omission of preventive actions, increased occurrence of chronic conditions, increased hospital visits, higher use of emergency services, and increased healthcare costs (ODPHP, 2017b). Although the responsibility to address and improve health literacy is shared, healthcare providers play a central role. One strategy for addressing the problems of poor health literacy is referred to as *plain language*, which is designed to use simple language and an active voice to organize information in understandable blocks with the most important content first.

SUMMARY

The imperative for students to learn clear communication skills in their courses is apparent. The need for good communication tools is broad and applies not only in education, but also in discussions, clinical conferences, and team meetings for patient care. We want to make communication as efficient and effective as possible. Communication tools will continue to evolve, and tools of lifelong learning will be needed to help gain strategies that best benefit our work with students. Good communication techniques are key in both creating a civil community of learners in our classrooms and for preparing our students to work on interprofessional clinical teams that provide safe, quality care.

ENDING REFLECTIONS FOR YOUR LEARNING NOTEBOOK

1. What is the most important content that you learned in this chapter?
2. What are your plans for using the information provided in this chapter in your future teaching endeavors?
3. What are your further learning goals?

GUIDELINES FOR TEACHING AND LEARNING WITH TECHNOLOGIES

Quick Teaching Tips

1. Remember the importance of introductions at the beginning of all classes to begin building the learning community (no matter what the technology focus of the course is).
2. Take the time early on to set the tone for frequent and friendly communications throughout the course. Use pictures of members of the learning community in courses where students are not seen to serve as a reminder of the human component.
3. Provide communication guides at the beginning of a course, telling students what to expect in respect to communication from you (e.g., response time for e-mail [within 24 hours], dates that you will be out of the office with limited e-mail access).
4. When writing a difficult e-mail to a student, have a trusted colleague read it for feedback and reread it a bit later yourself (or, preferably, both) before sending it.

Questions for Further Reflection

1. In what ways can technology be used to help promote clear, consistent communication between students and faculty?
2. In what ways can technology be used to help promote clear communication for patient care safety in the clinical setting?
3. What are your own strengths and weaknesses regarding respectful communication in the various aspects of your personal and professional life?

Learning Activity: Writing Exercises

Writing activities are versatile and lend themselves to a variety of feedback options, all of which encourage the development of critical thinking skills in students. Looking at the list of writing-to-learn activities below, challenge yourself to add as many new ideas as you can (add three at first, and then increase that by increments of three each time you succeed):

1. Write a focused summary of the day's reading assignment.
2. Identify a problem statement for the day's topic.
3. Write a letter to another student about the topic.

4. Write a project notebook.
5. Write a journal about the topic.
6. Write either a response paper or a synthesis paper.
7. End the session with a 5-minute writing exercise about what was learned that day (the main idea).

Online Resources for Further Learning

- University of Virginia, Teaching Resource Center. This site provides links to numerous teaching tips that transcend the technology used, including writing. cte.virginia.edu/resources/
- National Communication Association. This site has several sections of relevance to teaching and learning, including "Education" and "Research" sections. www.natcom.org

REFERENCES

Agency for Healthcare Research and Quality. (2016). Pocket guide: TeamSTEPPS. Retrieved from https://www.ahrq.gov/teamstepps/instructor/essentials/pocketguide.html
Arora, V., Gangireddy, S., Mehrotra, A., Ginde, R., Tormey, M., & Meltzer, D. (2009). Research letters. *JAMA Internal Medicine, 169*(2), 199–205. doi:10.1001/archinternmed.2008.565
Bonnel, W., Ludwig, C., & Smith, J. (2007). Providing feedback in online courses: What do students want? How do we do that? *Annual Review of Nursing Education, 6*, 205–221.
Clark, C. M. (2017). An evidence-based approach to integrate civility, professionalism, and ethical practice into nursing curricula. *Nurse Educator, 42*(3), 120–126. doi:10.1097/NNE.0000000000000331
Clark, C. M., & Springer, P. J. (2010). Academic nurse leaders' role in fostering a culture of civility in nursing education. *Journal of Nursing Education, 49*(6), 319–325. doi:10.3928/01484834-20100224-01
Dunn, E. J., Mills, P. D., Neily, J., Crittenden, M. D., Carmack, A. L., & Bagian, J. P. (2007). Medical team training: Applying crew resource management in the Veterans Health Administration. *Joint Commission Journal on Quality and Patient Safety, 33*(6), 317–325.
Eduscapes. (2008a). Teaching and learning at a distance, course communication. Retrieved from http://eduscapes.com/distance/course_communication/index.htm
Eduscapes. (2008b). Teaching and learning at a distance, course discussion: Prompts. Retrieved from http://eduscapes.com/distance/course_discussion/prompts.htm
Engard, B. (2016). The new netiquette: Internet etiquette in a modern world. Retrieved from https://online.philau.edu/communications/new-netiquette
Finkelman, A., & Kenner, C. (2014). *Teaching IOM: Implications of the Institute of Medicine reports for nursing education* (2nd ed.). Silver Spring, MD: American Nurses Association.
Gooch, K. (2016). The chronic problem of communication: Why it's a patient safety issue, and how hospitals can address it. Retrieved from https://www.beckershospitalreview.com/quality/the-chronic-problem-of-communication-why-it-s-a-patient-safety-issue-and-how-hospitals-can-address-it.html
Institute for Healthcare Communication. (2011). Impact of communication in healthcare. Retrieved from http://healthcarecomm.org/about-us/impact-of-communication-in-healthcare
Interprofessional Education Collaborative. (2016). *Core competencies for interprofessional collaborative practice: 2016 update*. Washington, DC: Author.
The Joint Commission. (2008). Behaviors that undermine a culture of safety. Retrieved from https://www.jointcommission.org/sentinel_event_alert_issue_40_behaviors_that_undermine_a_culture_of_safety
The Joint Commission. (2017). Speak up. Retrieved from https://www.jointcommission.org/speakup.aspx
National Assessment of Adult Literacy. (2006). The health literacy of America's adults. Retrieved from https://nces.ed.gov/pubsearch/pubsinfo.asp?pubid=2006483
National Communication Association. (2009). Communication defined. Retrieved from http://www.natcom.org/index.asp?bid=1339
Office of Disease Prevention and Health Promotion. (2017a). Fact sheet: Health literacy basics. Retrieved from https://health.gov/communication/literacy/quickguide/factsbasic.htm

Office of Disease Prevention and Health Promotion. (2017b). Fact sheet: Health literacy and health outcomes. Retrieved from https://health.gov/communication/literacy/quickguide/factsliteracy.htm

Polished. (2017). Seven must-know netiquette rules for professional behavior. Retrieved from https://stlpolished.com/seven-must-know-netiquette-rules-for-professional-behavior

Quality and Safety Education for Nurses Institute. (2017). QSEN competencies. Retrieved from http://qsen.org/competencies

Shea, V. (1994). *Netiquette*. San Francisco, CA: Albion Books.

Skiba, D. J., Connors, H. R., & Jeffries, P. R. (2009). Information technologies and the transformation of nursing education. *Nursing Outlook, 56*(5), 225–230. doi:10.1016/j.outlook.2008.06.012

Whaley, M. P. (2013). Can patient safety be improved by asking three questions? Retrieved from http://managemypractice.com/can-patient-safety-be-improved-by-asking-three-questions

Technology, Social Spaces, and Teaching and Learning Strategies to Build the Learning Community

CHAPTER GOAL

Gain tools for helping the learning community as a group to accomplish common learning goals.

BEGINNING REFLECTION

1. What is your definition of a learning community? How do the concepts of social learning and social media fit this definition?
2. What are the best teaching and learning experiences you have gained from participating in an online learning experience such as a discussion board?
3. What goals do you have for developing social learning assignments and facilitating learning communities?

Overheard: *I am not sure about this social media thing. I wish I could just ignore it.*

Learning is often considered a social activity. The need for contribution and relationships in learning as well as the important aspect of social and emotional learning are well noted (Carnegie Mellon University, 2015). In learning communities, course members bring diverse perspectives for learning together and can enhance learning for all. Learning communities provide opportunities for collaborative problem solving, a sense of connection, and acknowledgment for contributions (Brookfield & Preskill, 2005). Although learning communities are not a new phenomenon, the popularity of online education has led to increased attention to this concept. This chapter describes the strategies that faculty can use to help diverse student communities learn with technology support.

In this text, learning communities are considered to be groups of people engaged in common learning goals. They benefit from mutual cooperation, personal support, and synergy of efforts. Palloff and Pratt (2004) note that the concept of a learning community relates to more than knowledge gain or sharing; rather, the concept relates to an entire culture of learning. They describe a web of learning that includes not only concepts of content and technology, but also student, peer, and faculty learning participation. This concept is extended to consider social media as a part of online social learning.

Although the concept of learning community is often used to describe online learning, the concept has relevance across a broad range of teaching settings. Learning communities also help to promote the social aspect of face-to-face learning. As students share with one another as members of learning communities, they contribute to and strengthen collegial learning, providing a different approach to gaining knowledge. In addition, being part of a learning community includes exhibiting professional responsibility and being a good course citizen. Technology is a tool for engaging student learning communities and promoting learning.

Some learning community connections and activities are stronger than others. Learning community activities vary from individuals coming together to create new projects that meet learning objectives or to learn by sharing diverse experiences. Although any classroom might be considered a learning community, classrooms with strong student interaction geared toward mutual learning goals most closely fit the descriptor. From a constructivist perspective, students within learning communities share their learning experience, and others benefit as well. Although many different purposes are noted in the following examples, all might be groups coming together for learning purposes, and any of the following might represent a learning community:

- Associate degree nursing students working in small groups to develop posters for their community college health fair
- A graduate student group that meets face-to-face for 2 days and then participates in an online listserv to share challenges and successes as they develop their skills on a clinical topical area
- Students working on a quality assurance project in a long-term care practicum to focus on preventing the spread of infection

Several concepts are somewhat related to but different from the concept of the learning community as addressed in this text. The concept of a learning organization, for example, relates specifically to learning that is organization based and consists of paid employees working in groups on specific organizational problems. The concept of learning community has also been used to describe students who live together in a university setting to foster learning goals. The concept of online social communities is also popular, but these entities relate more to interactions and social networking than to learning tasks. These concepts and descriptors are not included in this discussion.

Learning communities can energize learning, moving learning from an isolated pursuit to a shared experience that helps students integrate concepts and make learning connections. Students learn to think about concepts differently as others share their experiences and examples. The example of differing approaches of two unique online geriatric courses conveys the concept of a learning community. In the first course, students write weekly papers, submit them to faculty for feedback, and receive a grade, all with total lack of knowledge of other students in the course. In the second course, students learn about each other's geriatric interests and goals for the course via introductory activities and a variety of assignments such as group activities, shared experiences, and topical discussions as the course progresses. Although approaches for each course might be justified, enormous learning opportunities are missed in the first course by not bringing the community together for learning.

Diverse student groups, learning purposes, and settings make each learning community unique. Settings for learning communities can vary from online classes to face-to-face classrooms, learning laboratories, and clinical settings. Learning communities can be directed toward learning content varying from obstetrics to long-term care of the older adult. Although this chapter focuses on the learning community in educational settings, faculty also want to prepare students for broad clinical learning communities that work together to solve clinical practice problems. Working as part of clinical teams is one of the recommendations of the health professions educator report (Institute of Medicine [IOM], 2003). Technologies such as those supporting online discussions provide unique opportunities for diverse health professions students to meet for interdisciplinary conversations. A goal in health professions education is to move education and practice closer together because we are preparing students to work together in healthcare organizations.

As students work together in learning communities, relationships between learners can be strengthened via community approaches to gaining knowledge. For example, one community approach is online discussions. These keep faculty easily apprised of students' experiences; students gain opportunity to compare their experiences with others'; and students learn and gain ideas/resources from one another that may have relevance at their own applied learning sites, providing a win-win situation.

Students gain focused opportunities to interact and participate in peer activities, learning together and providing feedback to one another. Feedback from faculty also connects learning community activities with furthering learning goals. Questions and challenges generate continued learning. Students maximize their learning by self-reflecting and conversing with others about the experiences in applied learning projects. Students often complete such at sites distant from one another, so there are benefits to moving their reflections and discussions about these experiences online. Faculty can provide direction in helping the learning community work together. Acknowledging diverse learners, considering their roles as community members, providing good direction, and facilitating students' work are important concepts. Principles of good group work based on systems theory provide the background for further discussion.

DIVERSE LEARNERS IN THE LEARNING COMMUNITY

Part of being a good teacher is knowing you have something new to learn about students at any given time and place (Bain, 2004). We find diversity in the classroom, in clinical settings, and in online courses. It is important to consider diverse students' needs not only to support learning together, but also to help them prepare for their future work as diverse clinicians working together in clinical settings. Group and team learning is an ongoing need in clinical settings (IOM, 2003).

Diverse students are good for a course. We seek to create a course that is good for diverse students. Human interactions make up all parts of our lives. Because learners are holistic beings, the social and emotional aspects of the classroom affect their learning (Carnegie Mellon University, 2015). Special attention is paid to group interactions. Concepts of collaboration and groups are key in course work that is centered around learning communities, allowing opportunities to learn from diverse learners.

A given technology may be less, or more, familiar to some populations because of cultural, age, and generational differences. Having a basic understanding of our students' backgrounds, interests, and educational attainment provides important context as we seek to move the learning community forward. Understanding the population provides direction in coaching and in providing optimal student learning resources.

Multigenerational Diversity

When we consider diversity, we need to consider how different generations come together and learn. Diverse generations of learners bring unique ways of being in the world. They bring different perspectives on what is important, how to learn, and how to work together. Diverse generations have learned in different ways with different tools. Groups that often need to learn and work together include the Millennials (those born in 1980s to early 1990s); Generation Xers (those born from the mid-1960s to late 1970s); and the aging Baby Boomers (those born 1940s to early 1960s) (Oblinger, 2003). For example, opportunities for students to participate in, interact with, experience, and construct knowledge to meet their own learning needs are consistent with learning styles of the new Millennial student generation but often vary from styles of other cohorts (Skiba, 2005). The unique needs and perspectives of each of these groups are worthy of attention when planning to teach with technologies.

Technologies and Diversity

We also see diversity in students' technology skills and enthusiasm for technology. Diverse generations have been described in various ways, including the net generation or digital natives, those who have grown up using technology, as distinguished from the non–net generation or digital immigrants, those who gain technology skills later in life (Skiba, 2005). The digital divide also describes the differences between those who have access to technology and those who do not (McGonigle & Mastrian, 2017).

Although access to technologies in the home setting has improved, faculty have a responsibility to provide alternative access methods if technology ownership is not a requirement of a program. Typically, there is more comfort with using technologies, but they can still be challenging for some learners, in particular the digital immigrants who find technologies a new way of doing things.

Cultural Diversity

Students making up our learning communities are becoming increasingly diverse, including not only diverse ethnic backgrounds, but also diverse socioeconomic backgrounds. These unique mixes of students can vary from those who are heads of households to those who are parent supported. Online education, in particular, has few geographic boundaries and has made programs more accessible, promoting opportunities for a larger pool of students to participate together. Diverse students bring unique background experiences and provide different perspectives on the larger world. Benefits include learning from a variety of perspectives as students young and old learn from one another's experiences and stories.

To work effectively with diverse students, we must understand the importance of broad definitions of diversity to fit our changing classrooms. Being mindful of the uniqueness of each student, being open-minded, and using diverse teaching strategies are good beginnings to try to meet a variety of learning needs. Ethical teaching principles described in early work by the American Association for Higher Education (Murray, Gillese, Lennon, Mercer, & Robinson, 1996) stress the importance of being sensitive to diverse student needs and preparing for and debriefing potentially difficult learning situations. A National League for Nursing (2015) publication on debriefing across the curriculum supports the ongoing importance of these concepts. Resources for helping faculty consider diversity are available, providing further ideas for thoughtful approaches to teaching and learning (Exhibit 7.1.)

BUILDING OUR LEARNING COMMUNITIES

Learning communities often complete work in groups. Nursing education and group assignments create an interesting mix. Putting students in groups does not automatically create collaboration. Group work has been described

EXHIBIT 7.1

RESOURCES FOR WORKING WITH DIVERSE STUDENTS

- "Diversity and Complexity in the Classroom." This chapter from the Barbara Gross Davis book, *Tools for Teaching*, provides a variety of practical strategies to work with a variety of diverse students, many of which can be applied to teaching and learning with technologies: cft.vanderbilt.edu/guides-sub-pages/diversity
- *Enhancing Diversity in the Nursing Workforce.* This resource summarizes current challenges in creating a diverse workforce and suggests strategies for enhancing diversity in both the classroom and the workplace: www.aacnnursing.org/News-Information/Fact-Sheets/Enhancing-Diversity

by numerous students as challenging. Examples of the challenges faced by groups of students, as reported in the literature, include unclear assignments, unwieldy group size, and social loafing (Kroen & Bonnel, 2007). Faculty members report their own challenges in facilitating online groups and grading group projects, such as clarifying group member project contributions.

Faculty take on roles as group facilitators in supporting the learning community. Group theory provides a broader background for working with learning communities, building on systems theory, and including concepts such as group development, group norms, and group structure and roles. Beginning considerations for successful groups, such as orientation, readiness for group activity, and peer evaluation, are provided in the literature (University of Sydney, n.d.). Fink (2013) notes that well-developed assignments and prompt feedback do much more to help teams improve their functioning than does teaching them about group interaction. Further tips for using groups effectively include promoting individual accountability and stimulating idea exchange with guiding questions. Group orientation guides and planning sheets for group members' roles, tasks, and specific outcomes provide good starting points for collaborative group work. Working as part of groups and teams is noted as preparation for important interprofessional teamwork in future clinical work (Interprofessional Education Collaborative, 2016).

Different needs are apparent at different points in the semester, so suggestions for each phase are outlined in the following sections. A focus on group beginnings, middles, and ends provides beginning direction in organizing work with our learning communities.

Beginnings

Course beginnings provide the opportunity to bring groups together with common interests and to help prepare students to be successful. Each unique student cohort brings fresh perspectives to learning at a given point in time. Technologies provide opportunities to help group members get to know one another. Introductory activities provide faculty, as well as students, with opportunities to learn about others and gain confidence in sharing. The diverse needs, abilities, and learning styles of each unique group can be ascertained to provide direction for guiding students in accomplishing learning goals. Suggested activities include the following.

GROUP INTRODUCTIONS AND SURVEYS OF THE CLASS

Whether prior to class or at the beginning of a classroom session, technologies provide opportunities to gain a quick snapshot of the students in the course, as well as to create opportunities for group connections. Group introductions and introductory surveys can highlight a group's characteristics, including basic demographic data such as age, background, and interests. In addition, reflective preclass questions can be generated that vary by topic studied. For example, asking students a very basic question about their experiences working with patients with Alzheimer's disease prior to a class on dementia serves as a type of assessment.

Depending on the setting, students can use e-mail, course management systems, or classroom clickers to complete these simple introductions and surveys. As students reflect and share, they begin to take more responsibility for learning, and faculty gain a better understanding of students' background and learning goals.

ORIENTING AND SETTING THE STAGE FOR THE LEARNING COMMUNITY

The beginning class session or module can be used to orient students to the workings and the value of being part of a learning community, as well as to create set, or context, for the class. A good student orientation includes an introduction to the learning community concept and the work of the class—not just the class content but the activities as well (Palloff & Pratt, 2004). Conveying the information that all students will be working together and gaining from one another's experiences and perspectives provides the beginning direction. Orientation can do the following:

- Convey benefits of active participation in learning
- Share guidelines for student responsibilities for participating in discussions and sharing with colleagues
- Provide tips for giving peer feedback (peer activities are particularly important ways to help students gain needed peer-review skills for the future)

Middles and Transitions

The goal of learning communities is to work together in learning, so assignments need to be designed to promote this outcome. As students are transitioning through often large amounts of information and projects, the possibility of losing momentum exists. The faculty facilitator role provides opportunities to help the class maintain momentum. Being proactive in assignment/course design and using good facilitator skills to engage with and encourage students promotes successful transitions throughout the assigned project or course.

PROVIDING ASSIGNMENTS THAT ALLOW MUTUAL LEARNING OPPORTUNITIES AND SHARING

Being proactive with good class design that engages learners promotes easier transitions and fewer challenges throughout a class session. Building in varied interaction modes helps meet diverse learner needs. If group projects are part of the class, guides include helping groups be clear on objectives, divide tasks, and determine what the final product will be. Peer review can be a component. Sharing of interviews or observations, work on team projects via portfolios, and discussions are useful tools in promoting group learning. Asking students to share experiences and perspectives promotes reflection, further learning, and relationships between learners; it also helps students gain perspectives on others' views of the world.

SERVING AS FACILITATOR FOR THE LEARNING COMMUNITY

Facilitating learning builds on good assignments and course design within a course focused on a student learning community. Facilitation includes faculty roles in engaging and encouraging students for ongoing learning within the community and assisting the community in accomplishing learning objectives. Students learn that faculty are present as course facilitators who promote group interactivity through the various group phases (Palloff & Pratt, 2004).

SYNTHESIZING AND SUMMARIZING

Faculty summarize and keep the community moving forward via feedback on discussions and shared activities. This ongoing/periodic feedback acknowledges emerging learning and connects activities with the goal of furthering learning. This includes reminding students of accomplishments to date and providing further questions and challenges that still need to be addressed.

Endings

Endings include reflection and debriefs as a group. These activities help students prepare for closure and further goal setting, whether at the conclusion of an assignment or the end of the semester.

BUILD IN REFLECTIVE OPPORTUNITIES

Sharing reflections about what has been learned via active class participation helps promote student learning. An isolated learning activity does not lead to understanding, but reflection on the activity itself helps promote understanding (Fink, 2013).

PROVIDE SYNTHESIS OF LEARNING ACCOMPLISHMENTS

Faculty can synthesize class accomplishments and relate these to overall class learning goals. This summary leads naturally to the "What next?" questions and can help students prepare for closure and further goal setting. For example, in an online class, a simple content analysis completed by faculty and an e-mail summary of key themes from web discussions provide the benefit of debriefing and providing feedback to students. Themes noted from discussions help summarize work and create links to past and future course content. Faculty serve as course guides in providing these summaries that also allow highlighting of discussion points, help students make conceptual connections from student examples, and bring closure to a topic.

Learning in Social Spaces

Online social spaces provide opportunities for student networking and assignments. Social media is considered technologies involved in sharing, exchanging, or creating ideas across networks. Schmitt, Sims-Giddens, and Booth (2012) indicate that the main use of social media is to engage others with web-based resources. These social networking sites engage friends or involve people who "follow" each other. As noted by the Pew Research Center (2017), Facebook is the most widely used social media platform and has a broad representative population, followed by Twitter, Pinterest, Instagram, and LinkedIn.

Social media is also a tool commonly used for professional communication. For example, professional networking and the ability to stay connected with followers has been reported by individuals as improved after the use of Twitter. Tweets or "shout outs" are a form of recreational microblogging, so all users are empowered for amateur journalism. The real value of Twitter is in limited character posts designed to stream quick updates for family, friends, scholars, and the world; in addition, hashtags can be used to find and follow tweets about a specific topic or theme. Using hand-held mobile devices, individuals can expeditiously share and learn "tweeting" in the most appropriate moment.

Responsible use of social media is part of being a professional, and challenges exist. With younger students, in particular, there seems to be challenges determining boundaries between professional and personal lives online. Understanding that nurses of 2025 will inhabit a practice environment transformed with technology (Risling, 2017), including advanced information and communication venues, it is particularly important to address a respectful professional environment.

Social media raises questions and issues related to social networking and professionalism (Prinz, 2001). This requires that educators maintain professional boundaries and guide students in maintaining a professional presence in all online venues. Knowing how to behave as a professional is guided by standards and codes of the profession. Resources, such as those developed by Centers for Disease Control and Prevention (n.d.), provide guidance in best communication practices for healthcare activities, campaigns, and emergency response efforts.

All programs need to have policies relevant to social media use. Standards of the profession serve as guides and resources to share with students. Appropriate guidance in developing policies can be gained from professional documents such as standards and scope of practice documents including diverse resources from organizations such as the American Nurses Association, the National Council of State Boards of Nursing, and the Technology Informatics Guiding Education

Reform (TIGER) initiative. Questions to ponder relevant to the use of social media include the following: What are potential issues or challenges (such as privacy and incivility)? How will these issues best be addressed? And will the social media application meet the Owens (2016) THINK standards (meaning, is it: T = true, H = helpful, I = inspiring, N = necessary, and K = kind).

BEING A GOOD COURSE CITIZEN: THE ETIQUETTE OF LEARNING TOGETHER WITH TECHNOLOGIES

In today's technology-rich classroom, both face-to-face and online civility and digital citizenship are important community concepts. Students take on community membership to some degree in all courses, regardless of the course type. Students learn that being good community members includes acknowledging professional roles and rules for good citizenship with technologies. Although relevant across all technologies, this topic is particularly important in online classrooms because there may be added challenges if face-to-face communication benefits are missing. The International Society for Technology in Education (2008) standards include three broad considerations related to learning together with technologies:

- Developing positive attitudes toward technology applications that support collaboration, lifelong learning, and productivity
- Understanding the ethical, cultural, and societal issues related to technologies
- Practicing responsible use of technology systems, information, and software

Although varied technologies present different citizenship issues, concepts of safety and security in the digital world are broadly applicable. Professional behaviors, including respectful awareness of all learning community members, are key factors. Faculty can be proactive with guidelines that promote good course citizenship and appropriate use of technologies for learning (rather than spending class time focused on problem solving when breeches occur). Besides providing students with an orientation to expected classroom roles, citizenship guides describing good citizenship standards can be provided. Ideas for developing guidelines for "digital citizenship" can be gained from a review of sample documents on the Internet. Depending on the level of the class, concepts may be as basic as being respectful of one another and being responsible in the use of technology. Asking students to complete a digital citizenship audit that includes self-assessments of personal technology behaviors has been recommended. (Ribble, Bailey, & Ross, 2004). General guidelines include the following:

- Take a prospective approach to developing a positive learning community.
- Orient students to school handbooks of professional conduct.

- Consider developing class civility documents.
- Ask students to sign technology codes of conduct that include broad guides for appropriate use of digital devices.

Professional communication in the clinical setting becomes even more complex with technologies such as text-based communication, including text messages. As health professionals, we also have professional ethical guidelines to meet. In nursing, for example, the American Nurses Association provides ethical guidelines that direct ethical behavior in the profession. Consequences to all professions can be major if we do not address important ethical issues. With rapidly changing technologies in the classroom, all the rules for good citizenship have not yet been developed. Ribble et al. (2004) suggest continued questioning of what is and is not an appropriate use of technology, anticipating that our descriptions of what is appropriate will change over time.

SUMMARY

Learning communities have goals of learning together. Teaching goals include providing diverse teaching and learning methods for diverse learners, as well as promoting professional, civic-minded learning communities. Attending to selected strategies with beginnings, transitions, and endings of course learning communities provides direction. As we prepare students for future clinical work, group learning situations provide practice for working in clinical teams. The varied settings in which our student learning communities will be expected to function provide impetus for our work. Learning communities can be powerful tools and take learning far beyond traditional classroom approaches.

ENDING REFLECTIONS FOR YOUR LEARNING NOTEBOOK

1. What is the most important content that you learned in this chapter?
2. What are your plans for using the information provided in this chapter in your future teaching endeavors?
3. What are your further learning goals?

GUIDELINES FOR TEACHING AND LEARNING WITH TECHNOLOGIES

Quick Teaching Tips

1. Acknowledge diverse learners. Recognize contributions of individuals and provide opportunities for individuals to participate in self-assessment and peer review.
2. Participate in the learning community, but do not dominate it. In the online setting, provide regular communications to affirm social presence.

3. Provide learning spaces, including online discussions and document sharing, for the community's work. This can be in the form of online discussion boards, Google Docs, or collaborative concept mapping tools.

Questions for Further Reflection

1. What learning community activities for a given topic would best promote students' learning together?
2. Although technology often helps us bring more diverse students to our classrooms, how do we most effectively meet these students' needs in our courses?
3. What issues related to the potential for inappropriate use of technology need to be considered in course learning communities?
4. What benefits and challenges do you identify in your nurse educator work with social spaces such as Facebook?

Learning Activity: Engaging Communities

Create an assignment: The purpose of this assignment is to engage learning community students in sharing a clinical topic important to them at a group blog. The activity might take a reflective writing approach, asking students to blog about a personal or family/client experience demonstrating issues related to family caregivers of those suffering from Alzheimer's disease. This personal experience could then be related to the broader literature and best-practice evidence. Group members gain learning and sharing opportunities at several levels.

Online Resources for Further Learning

- Social Media Guidelines for Nurses (provided by the NCSBN in both print and video format). This resource review helps you gain ideas and resources for ongoing and future work. www.ncsbn.org/347.htm
- Google Docs: an online platform where users can write, edit, and collaborate anytime using a computer or phone. www.google.com/docs/about/
- Sharing Mayo Clinic. This resource provides a clinical employee guide to social media use relevant to the clinical work setting. sharing.mayoclinic .org/guidelines/for-mayo-clinic-employees

REFERENCES

Bain, K. (2004). *What the best college teachers do*. Cambridge, MA: Harvard University Press.

Brookfield, S. D., & Preskill, S. (2005). *Discussions as a way of teaching: Tools and techniques for democratic classrooms* (2nd ed.). San Francisco, CA: Jossey-Bass.

Carnegie Mellon University. (2015). Principles of learning. Retrieved from https://www.cmu.edu/teaching/principles/learning.html

Centers for Disease Control and Prevention. (2018). U.S. Department of Health & Human Services. Retrieved from https://www.cdc.gov/

Fink, L. D. (2013). *Creating significant learning experiences: An integrated approach to designing college courses*. San Francisco, CA: Jossey-Bass.

Institute of Medicine. (2003). *Health professions education: A bridge to quality*. Washington, DC: National Academies Press.

International Society for Technology in Education. (2008). The national educational technology standards and performance indicators for teachers. Retrieved from https://www.iste.org/docs/pdfs/20-14_ISTE_Standards-T_PDF.pdf

Interprofessional Education Collaborative. (2016). *Core competencies for interprofessional collaborative practice: 2016 update*. Washington, DC: Author.

Kroen, K., & Bonnel, W. (2007, February). *Applied learning, group assignments and online courses: Toward developing best practices*. Conference on Applied Learning in Higher Education, St. Joseph, MO.

McGonigle, D., & Mastrian, K. (2017). *Nursing informatics and the foundation of knowledge. Informatics for health professionals*. Boston, MA: Jones & Bartlett.

Murray, H., Gillese, E., Lennon, M., Mercer, P., & Robinson, M. (1996). American Association for Higher Education bulletin. Retrieved from https://www.aahea.org/articles/Ethical+Principles.htm

National Council of State Boards of Nursing. (2011). White paper: A nurse's guide to the use of social media. Retrieved from https://www.ncsbn.org/Social_Media.pdf

National League for Nursing. (2015). Debriefing across the curriculum. Retrieved from http://www.nln.org/docs/default-source/about/nln-vision-series-(position-statements)/nln-vision-debriefing-across-the-curriculum.pdf?sfvrsn=0

Oblinger, D. (2003). Boomers, Gen-Xers, Millennials: Understanding the new students. *Educause Review, 38*, 37–47.

Owens, J. K. (2016). Posting on social media. Retrieved from http://naepub.com/social-media/2016-26-1-5

Palloff, R. M., & Pratt, K. (2004). *Collaborating online: Learning together in community*. San Francisco, CA: Jossey-Bass.

Pew Research Center. (2017). Social media fact sheet. Retrieved from http://www.pewinternet.org/fact-sheet/social-media

Prinz, A. (2011). Professional social networking for nurses. *American Nurse Today*. Retrieved from https://www.americannursetoday.com/professional-social-networking-for-nurses

Ribble, M., Bailey, G., & Ross, T. (2004). Digital citizenship, addressing appropriate technology behavior. *Learning and Leading with Technology, 32*(1), 6–11.

Risling, T. (2017). Educating the nurses of 2025: Technology trends of the next decade. *Nurse Education in Practice, 22*, 89–92. doi:10.1016/j.nepr.2016.12.007

Schmitt, T. L., Sims-Giddens, S. S., & Booth, R. G. (2012). Social media use in nursing education. *Online Journal of Issues in Nursing, 17*(3), 2.

Skiba, D. J. (2005). The Millennials: Have they arrived at your school of nursing? *Nursing Education Perspectives, 26*(6), 370–371.

The University of Sydney School of Education and Social Work. (2018). Learning and teaching group work guide for staff and students. Retrieved from http://sydney.edu.au/education_social_work/groupwork

CHAPTER 8

Applied Technologies Assignments: Engaging the Learner for Quality and Safety

CHAPTER GOAL

Gain resources and strategies for making active learning an integral part of a teaching toolbox.

BEGINNING REFLECTION

1. In what ways do you incorporate the science of learning into your teaching strategies?
2. What experiences have you had that relate to creating active learning assignments to enhance quality and safety?
3. What ideas do you have for assignments for which you might incorporate active learning?

Overheard: *All this reading just seems like looking at a wall of words. What am I supposed to do with all this?*

Learning is complex in today's technology-rich world. Technology has made it much easier to deliver learning activities and assignments to students. Active learning with technologies provides students with the opportunity to integrate real-world experiences into virtual or face-to-face class experiences, providing opportunity to truly experience course content. As students prepare to provide safe, quality care in the clinical setting, active learning with technologies that prepare them for this role are particularly important.

This chapter focuses on making learning real and active, considering technology as a tool for promoting active learning. Appropriate for either traditional classroom teaching or online courses, technology-supported active learning assignments can be timely, efficient approaches for teaching and enhancing student learning. Opportunity for creativity in using technology as a part of active learning assignments abounds. Fink (2013) noted that one of the most important things faculty can do to promote learning is expand active learning activities.

ACTIVE LEARNING AND THE SCIENCE OF LEARNING

The science of learning has gained increasing interests and guides us in focusing on not only traditional teaching strategies alone, but also those strategies that best help students learn (Ambrose, Bridges, DiPietro, Lovett, & Norman, 2010; Brown, Roediger, & McDaniel, 2014; National Academy of Sciences [NAS], 2015). For example, key points in helping students learn include becoming intentional learners, framing and solving problems, and practicing and gaining authentic experience (NAS, 2015). These concepts, consistent with active learning, also fit well with strategies to promote student learning for safe, quality care. Part of the educator role is creating significant learning opportunities for students to be successful (Fink, 2013). Educators are encouraged to consider these points as they read this chapter and develop assignment plans for students.

WHAT ARE ACTIVE LEARNING ASSIGNMENTS?

Assignments are considered any activities that help students learn or that assess student learning. Assignments or strategies that incorporate writing, reflecting, or quizzing are examples. These activities provide an opportunity to apply content for practice and learning. Assignments serve as tools to help students focus on concepts, helping them better understand and use new information in meaningful ways. Student skill sets are developed via well-designed assignments based on learning objectives.

Adult education theory (Knowles, 1984) posits that students learn by applying concepts in meaningful ways. Active learning engages students in doing something with the content that is being taught. Brookfield and Preskill (2005) describe the importance of engaging the body and the mind in learning. In contrast to more traditional lecture formats, faculty can engage students and extend their knowledge of course content using varied technologies. In an active learning mode, students gain information, do something with the information, and then reflect on what has been learned. Students miss real-world applications if they only sit and listen to classroom presentations or just read and answer basic factual study questions to complete online courses.

Although a clinical practice component is an expected part of student learning in nursing programs, some faculty may be more comfortable with classroom teaching and traditional evaluation methods of testing. The idea of active learning that helps students directly apply content with impact for safe, quality patient care may not initially be comfortable. Doing something with specified content gives students practice in synthesizing knowledge and skills in preparation for the complex tasks they will complete in clinical settings. When learning how to do otoscopic examinations, for example, students can read about the topic and observe practitioners, but often it is not until they actively practice or apply the strategy in the clinical laboratory or with patients that the concepts make sense. Although we want students to read and understand key information, it is more likely they will understand and recall the concepts if they apply the concepts via projects of some type. Often it is not until students are working on assigned projects that key points come together. Active learning strategies can range from discussion questions to role-playing to virtual tours. Technology makes active learning tools—from flashcards to question-and-answer games or automated quizzes—all more accessible.

Active learning carries through the theme of helping students learn how to learn; students gain practice in active situations that help them transition to practice. Students also gain skills for lifelong learning. Various concepts related to active learning have related or similar meanings. The terms *active learning, authentic learning, applied learning, and experiential learning* are often used in close association. Each term describes opportunities for students to apply knowledge and skills in an immediate and relevant setting (Knowles, 1984). For our purposes, we use the following broad descriptors.

- **Active learning**. *Active learning* will be considered the broader term in this discussion. It refers to using or doing something with information gained. Information would be gained from a reading, for example, and then applied via some type of activity or assignment. Active learning makes the connection between the facts presented and actual clinical application (Fink, 2013).
- **Authentic learning**. Authentic learning occurs when active strategies are used to engage in realistic activities or develop projects with relevance to a real need.
- **Applied learning**. Applied learning is beneficial in reminding us to take information gained in the classroom to the clinical or community setting (a common approach in health professions education).
- **Experiential learning**. Experiential learning is considered learning around experiences, including direct participation in specific activities. Students reflect and gain meaning.

Teaching approaches that make learning real and active are used in each context to meet diverse learner needs. Within each approach, students gain the opportunity to be more engaged in learning. For the purposes of our discussion, terms are grouped under the concepts of active learning. Technology provides opportunities to make teaching and learning more active.

WHAT ARE BEST PRACTICES RELATED TO ACTIVE LEARNING?

Active learning is consistent with a variety of theories and best practices. Examples include the following:

- **Adult learning theory** (Knowles, 1984). Adult learning theory reminds us to ask, when developing lesson plans, how we can build on students' current knowledge/experience, make the content relevant to students, and help them apply that content.

- **Constructivist learning theory.** Constructivism reminds us to provide assignments that are useful to students in constructing their own learning and understanding.
- **Principles for good practices in teaching.** The Chickering and Gamson (1987) classic reference includes seven research-supported principles for undergraduate education, including a focus on using active learning techniques that respect diverse learners' talents and ways of learning.
- **Principles of learning.** Research-supported learning principles, consistent with active learning, include building on content learning, combining and integrating content with practice, and understanding when to apply content learned (Carnegie Mellon University, 2015; NAS, 2015).

TECHNOLOGY AND ACTIVE LEARNING: AUDIO AND VISUAL EXAMPLES

Applied, active learning strategies synthesize much learning evidence. In addition, helping students become intentional learners is consistent across evidence summaries (Ambrose et al., 2010; Brown et al., 2014; NAS, 2015). Optimizing audio and visual technologies can begin to help students focus their learning and apply this knowledge actively. Irrespective of whether our teaching is online, face-to-face, or in a clinical setting, a key concept includes making a good fit between the learning we want for students and the assignments and technology tools that we choose for our classes. Providing students with a variety of assignment types helps meet the needs of diverse learners. Although listening to an audio presentation or watching a video provides learning opportunities, these activities are often completed while doing something else or multitasking. Technology provides opportunities to engage diverse learners who bring diverse learning styles to class. Auditory, visual, and kinesthetic learning styles can all be enhanced by a variety of technology-supported assignments.

Active Auditory Learning

Listening has long been a component of learning. Intonation is part of our language and provides cues to meaning. We use verbal cues in many ways in the classroom, such as accepting and reacting to student emotions, providing positive reinforcement, giving appropriate classroom feedback to students, using questioning as a tool, giving information, and giving direction. We also use nonverbal cues in the classroom, such as eye contact, gestures, mannerisms, movement, facial expressions, posture, energy level, and use of space. When audio becomes the focus, the educator is challenged to make the audio presentation to the point, interesting, and engaging.

In the authors' early graduate school years, listening to audio tapes while driving seemed a good use of time. MP3 players such as iPods have since taken their place and bring even more flexibility to learning on the run. Podcasts have made learning on the go a popular feature, highlighting interest in audio learning. Faculty are accessing or creating podcasts of lectures and delivering these to students via web venues. The VARK (visual, aural, read/write, kinesthetic) learning inventory and learning style modalities provide additional opportunity for assignments, asking students to, for example, complete the VARK inventory and consider their best learning modes (VARK Learn, 2017).

In addition, tools, including voice-over PowerPoint presentations and classroom capture tools such as Camtasia, expand and provide enhanced audio learning opportunities. Tools such as Adobe web conferencing add an interactive audio component to web-based learning. Although these technologies provide teaching and learning opportunities, best practices need to be considered in their implementation.

How can audio be used as active learning? In considering how best to use podcasts, faculty might listen to a podcast, via The Podcasting Group, to a 30-minute podcast, and then ask three questions:

- How much of the material did I retain?
- Did I focus the entire time on the podcast (or was I multitasking in a way that prevented engaging in the learning)?
- What other ways do I think the content might have been presented to better engage the learner?

As noted, asking learners to do something with the information helps keep them engaged. This strategy can be as basic as asking learners to complete a worksheet based on the audio session or reflecting on specified questions.

Active Visual or Video Learning

Visual images can help convey key points and place learning in context. For example, simple diagrams can help students recall complex anatomy or physiology concepts and more easily place content in context. Visual learners benefit from a variety of visual learning tools such as flowcharts, graphs, and colors. The VARK learning inventory and learning style modalities, as noted, provide additional opportunity for student assignments such as assessments and discussions about multimodal approaches (VARK Learn, 2017).

Benefits of using videos include convenience for students, potential for active learning when used correctly, benefits of demonstrating content, access to real-life cases/interviews, and potential for reruns/reviews that can benefit the student. Just being able to stop and start the video at convenient times allows opportunity to discuss topics in class or to replay key points.

Videos also make us observers and can serve many purposes in teaching and learning. They can help create context for learning when clinical settings become part of the video, depicting, for example, very personal patient situations or critical care situations that would be hard for large student numbers to observe in real time. For example, providing students a video tour of the operating room before clinical experiences may promote an easier transition to this setting and make the tour accessible to increased numbers of students. Faculty play important roles in setting the learning stage for video and debriefing the experience, whether face-to-face or online.

Concepts and boundaries of video are blurring. Videos are shown in face-to-face classrooms, on computer-based DVDs, or as web-based scenarios. Video applications have recently included streaming video (video on the Internet), instructional televised video in the classroom via a two-way interactive connection, one-way live video to the classroom with opportunity for call-in questions, podcasts, and compact disc–based videos (CD-ROM). Video for the traditional classroom, such as resources from the Public Broadcasting System, are also available.

Faculty roles with a video presentation include much more than just clicking a link for student viewing. The same teaching–learning concepts of engaging students apply across a variety of video types. Relevant to active learning, we ask students to do something with the video content. For example, the faculty might provide discussion prompts or questions for students to think about while watching the video. In some ways this is similar to further developing guideline s for a reflective observer role. We want students to think about what they are viewing and what they will do with this information. Chapter 14 further addresses the observer role.

Although our discussion does not relate to major video production, broad guidelines can help avoid "talking heads" or the "snooze factor" that prevail in some videos. Further tips for audiovisual teaching and learning are provided by diverse web resources such as the Information and Communication Technology (ICT) Across the Curriculum blog (ictacrossthecurriculum .wordpress.com/about). If you are assigning a specific audio or video activity, sample tips for engaging students for audio and video learning (synchronous or asynchronous) include the following:

- Orient or prepare students for what is going to be happening (create set either verbally or by written notation).
- Incorporate active learning (some strategy for interacting with the video content such as questions to answer or worksheets as before-and-after activities).
- Provide opportunities to discuss and debrief the learning points from the video.

If you are presenting content via a video presentation:

- Avoid being a talking head. Incorporate engaging prompts or questions for student reflection.
- Be prepared for presentations to avoid the distraction of shuffled papers.
- Be aware of your nonverbal motions and consider whether they distract from the message (completing a self-assessment on a video of your own teaching can be useful).

Challenges in Audiovisual Learning

Although there are many benefits of audiovisual learning, there are also challenges to consider. What are our roles as providers of audiovisual materials, for example, with the following issues?

- Great variability exists in the quality of audio and video materials available. What is our faculty role in critiquing these tools before sharing them with students?
- What is the faculty role in production? Should faculty create videos? How professional do these videos need to be? What resources are available? Does something available already capture the desired teaching concepts? A fair amount of time, energy, and resources go into completing a professional-quality video. It is also harder to make changes to a video than to a web page.
- What are the issues when students seek their own online videos as learning tools? What types of review criteria should students have for choosing online videos to watch?
- What are the benefits and challenges of assignments in which students create their own videos?

ACTIVE LEARNING MODES: AUTHENTIC ASSIGNMENTS

Gaining authentic experience is an important learning concept. Putting learning into context, whether online or face-to-face, helps students gain a more authentic experience, which can assist them in making sense of new material and recalling it later (Fink, 2013; NAS, 2015). Isolated facts are easily forgotten, and context created by faculty helps students make sense of information. Strategies for expanding our toolbox of active learning strategies fall into the following broad categories: stories, cases, interviews, and observations. Even though we are using technologies, we are back to the basics of familiar tools/concepts and good educational principles.

Stories and Cases

Stories help students move from a simple listing of facts to application via story. Consistent with constructivism models, learning involves making or constructing meaning as stories allow one to do (Szurmak & Thuna, 2013). Stories allow the big picture of a problem or situation to emerge, providing not only facts, but also the context for the facts. A single story or case can meet multiple learning purposes. Stories and cases are closely related concepts, with stories providing a more descriptive, narrative approach and cases a more detailed factual approach. Both provide opportunities to share examples in a nonthreatening way that promotes opportunity for thought and discussion. These tools can provide either an introduction to or a reinforcement of a topic area. Stories can bring a more humanistic component to teaching with technologies. Stories and cases help faculty accomplish the following goals:

- Provide the connection between the textbook and the lived experience, making concepts more easily memorable.
- Relate new concepts to other, more familiar concepts.
- Show how concepts can be applied in similar ways across different populations or settings, extending understandings about certain illnesses. For example, a scenario could be provided of two different patients, one with early Parkinson's disease and one with late-stage Parkinson's disease.

Problem-based learning, incorporating the concept of ongoing expanding stories or cases, is another related concept with benefits of case sharing. Today's technologies allow stories to be shared in new and important ways, as described in Exhibit 8.2 at the end of the chapter.

Interview and Observation Assignments

Authentic assignments that engage students with real-world experiences provide another opportunity for expanding learning with technology. These authentic assignments provide students with opportunities to learn from experts on selected topics and gain real-world perspectives. Student reflections and summaries can be shared with the learning community to extend perspectives on a topic. By completing interview assignments with professionals working in a specialty clinical area, for example, students can learn and gain knowledge from these experts. This activity also provides students opportunities to seek and gain mentors.

Developing observation assignments for students, whether direct observation or participant observation, provides students opportunity to add real-world perspective to class concepts. Students learning about group theory, for example, might observe a community-based group education session or support group. Further ideas for engaging students with interviews and observations are provided by Bonnel and Meek (2007).

CREATING MEANINGFUL ASSIGNMENTS

All assignments are not created equal. What makes one assignment better than another? How do we creatively put together interesting learning activities for our students? Rather than asking "What should I cover in this class," asking "What should my students learn to do" provides more direction. Walvoord and Anderson (2009) describe concepts of fit and feasibility in assignment design. Focusing on the "doing" component of learning can guide assignment development.

Particularly with text-based communication, we want clear, accessible guidelines. These guidelines include being clear as to whether the assignment supports ongoing learning or serves as part of a final grade. The concepts of formative and summative evaluation are discussed further in Chapter 9. Developing a course assignment map of when and where assignments exist in the semester can be useful (Walvoord & Anderson, 2009). This approach also helps to see whether assignments fit course goals and whether these assignments are manageable in terms of workload. This map helps develop an assignment-centered course with focus on outcomes rather than content. Building on concepts within the Integrated Learning Triangle for Teaching With Technologies (Exhibit 1.3) provides direction. Sample points to consider in writing an assignment include the following:

- Consider the context. What is the context for this assignment? Who are the students? What type of course will this assignment be incorporated into?
- Include a strong purpose statement. What is the point of this assignment? How will completing this assignment help students prepare for current or future practice? How will this activity help students learn? Including an assignment introduction helps students understand the major intent of the assignment and lets them know what is in it for them.
- Determine your objectives for the assignment. Specific assignment objectives lay the framework for assignment evaluation. Questions to guide objectives development include the following: What is the point of this assignment? How will this activity help students engage in active learning? How does this activity help students improve their critical thinking?
- Use activities that actively engage students with using the content. As noted earlier, active engagement promotes students in learning and promotes critical thinking.
- Name assignments to help convey the intended learning goals. A good assignment name used consistently also helps avoid confusion when communicating with students.
- Provide clear directions. Particularly with text-based communication that lacks immediate opportunities for clarification, potential for student confusion in reading directions exists. Although our guidelines can seem fairly clear to us, usually we can benefit from having additional readers give feedback as to their clarity.

Reflection as Added Value for Assignments

Self-reflection provides additional opportunity for interaction with the content. As students reflect on an assignment, they gain an opportunity to build on their past experiences and incorporate current learning experiences. Irrespective of whether online or in-class, Fink (2013) has noted that one relatively easy way to both engage students and extend learning includes asking them to complete more self-reflections.

For example, self-reflection against an assignment rubric helps students gain skills in judging the quality of their work, judging their self-knowledge, and determining when more learning is needed. Billings (2005) noted that self-reflection helps students learn how to transfer concepts from theory to practice and from one context to another. Reflection provides an opportunity to think about learning from one's experience and leads to self-directed learning. Providing benchmark indicators via rubrics and asking students to identify how they have accomplished them help gain student perceptions of outcomes.

Assignment Repositories

Many electronic repositories of useful resources and assignments are being developed for teaching students across a variety of settings. These sites for gathering electronic documents and resources for teaching and learning provide a win-win situation, often supplying active learning assignment ideas for faculty. The Quality and Safety Education for Nurses (QSEN) Institute, for example, focuses on resources and assignments that can help students gain recommended health professions competencies. Opportunities exist for others to use these assignments, further evaluate them, and then share them with others. Peer-review opportunities exist as part of many of these repositories to assist in further developing the best teaching strategies. They also serve as an opportunity for peer review to promote scholarship with our teaching. Sample resources are provided in Exhibit 8.1.

In addition, student textbooks often have accompanying faculty and student guides either in electronic or hard-copy format. Although these resources vary in depth, many of the assignment suggestions can easily be adapted to fit specific course needs and technologies.

As discussed earlier, an evidence-based review abstract about storytelling is provided in Exhibit 8.2. This synthesis of best evidence provides further direction for our work as educators.

EXHIBIT 8.1

ELECTRONIC REPOSITORIES

Sample repositories providing resources for active learning assignments can be found at the following websites:

- QSEN Institute: www.qsen.org
- Multimedia Educational Resource for Learning and Online Teaching: www.merlot.org/merlot/index.htm
- MIT OpenCourseWare: ocw.mit.edu
- MedEdPORTAL: www.aamc.org/mededportal
- The HEAL: www.healcentral.org

HEAL, Health Education Assets Library; MIT, Massachusetts Institute of Technology; QSEN, Quality and Safety Education for Nurses.

EXHIBIT 8.2

EVIDENCE-BASED REVIEW ABSTRACT: STORYTELLING AS A TEACHING AND LEARNING CONCEPT

Compiled by: Cheryl A. Spittler, PhD, RN, CPSN

The following summary provides a graduate student's experience of synthesizing literature for her work in helping cancer patients better understand clinical options via stories from others.

Storytelling has been around since the beginning of time and is a way to learn history and communicate information; it can be viewed as a form of entertainment. It is a familiar way of relating information and can provide knowledge on different topics. A systematic literature review identified that both qualitative and quantitative researchers have found that evidence-based practice exists for storytelling. Storytelling is an inexpensive teaching method and can be used to understand the meaning of an experience and improve the process of learning. Possible benefits of telling a story are to express information uniquely, aid in problem solving, provide diversity in the ways of knowing, make learning more memorable, and contribute to another way of knowing. In regard to patient education, stories may help people gain confidence with procedures, acquire skills quicker, decrease stress, aid in patient–family trust development, and improve memory retention.

In addition, storytelling may lead to further truths on different topics and help patients understand the meaning of experiences in a better way. A model case was developed of storytelling as a teaching and learning concept for use with a group of women diagnosed with breast cancer. Listening to podcasts with other cancer survivor testimonies is a way to use storytelling to convey important information such as treatment options and decisions, personal experiences, frequently encountered problems and concerns, and knowing how to access available support services. Technology serves as a tool for conveying the stories. Further research specific to combining storytelling with technologies is recommended.

SUMMARY

Consistent with evidence from the science of teaching and learning, technology provides an opportunity to increase active learning for our students, making learning real and authentic. The types of learning activities we provide help students gain skills for their future professional practice. Both the QSEN Institute (2017) and the Health Professions Education report (Institute of Medicine, 2003) emphasize incorporating technology into curricula as a high-priority competency. A variety of assignments help meet students' diverse learning needs and prepare students for practice. Active learning, including audio and visual learning modes, as well as authentic assignments such as interviews and observations, provides tools for engaging students for learning.

ENDING REFLECTIONS FOR YOUR LEARNING NOTEBOOK

1. What is the most important content that you learned in this chapter?
2. What are your plans for using the information provided in this chapter in your future teaching endeavors?
3. What are your further learning goals?

GUIDELINES FOR TEACHING AND LEARNING WITH TECHNOLOGIES

Quick Teaching Tips

1. Use a variety of technology-based mediums, such as audio, video, and applied learning to meet diverse learners' needs.
2. Engage students by sharing authentic applied learning activities and assignments.
3. Provide relevant student assignments with clear purpose statements and guidelines.
4. Provide opportunities for learners to reflect and share their stories (or experiences) and build on these stories in teaching and learning sessions.
5. Become familiar with electronic learning resources and repositories to enhance teaching with technologies opportunities.

Questions for Further Reflection

1. What ways can audiovisuals be presented to best engage our students?
2. What are the benefits and challenges of synchronous versus asynchronous uses of audiovisual learning?
3. In what ways can audiovisual materials help extend a meaningful faculty presence?

Learning Activity: Technology Interview

Select someone in your nursing school or healthcare agency who has experience in teaching with a selected technology. Ask if this individual, in the spirit of knowledge sharing, would be willing to talk with you about personal experiences teaching with a particular technology. Sample questions might include the following:

1. What types of students and courses do you use this technology with?
2. What do you like about teaching with this technology?
3. Is there a particular assignment you like for engaging students and promoting active learning?
4. What were some of the challenges for you in getting started teaching with this technology? What have been some of the positive outcomes you have seen?
5. What advice do you have for a new faculty member beginning work in teaching with this technology?

Learning Activity: Create an Assignment

SAMPLE ASSIGNMENT—GLOBAL POPULATION HEALTH AND THE INTERNET

The purpose of this type of assignment is to help students gain quality nursing resources for promoting health or addressing need from local to international venues. Varied Internet resources can serve as resources for educational tools or evidence-based protocols for nurses providing care across a state, a country, or the world. Use the following concepts to write an assignment for relevance to students.

Ask students to create a document that involves identifying a quality website that can be used to gain guidance regarding a health issue in a select population. Population need and rationale for the selected website should be provided. For example, sample web resources could include the Centers for Disease Control and Prevention (CDC), the World Health Organization (WHO), or the American Red Cross. Students critique the website in terms of usefulness for nurses dealing with select populations. They are also asked to identify practical opportunities for using the web resource in practice.

Online Resources for Further Learning

The purpose of this resource review is to help you gain ideas and resources for ongoing and future work. The following have particular reference in guiding ongoing development of active learning approaches with technologies.

- Critical Thinking, Key Concepts (select from the Library/Articles section). This resource provides further review and teaching tips for developing critical thinking from the Center for Critical Thinking. www.criticalthinking.org
- Teaching Tools and Techniques, Techniques for Student Engagement and Classroom Management in Large (and Small) Classes. This resource on engaging students is provided by the National Teaching and Learning Forum. www.ntlf.com/html/lib/suppmat/teachingtools.pdf

REFERENCES

Ambrose, S. A., Bridges, M. W., DiPietro, M., Lovett, M. C., & Norman, M. K. (2010). *How learning works: Seven research-based principles*. San Francisco, CA: Jossey-Bass.

Billings, D. (2005). Teaching for higher order learning. *Journal of Continuing Education in Nursing, 36*(6), 244–245. doi:10.3928/0022-0124-20051101-03

Bonnel, W., & Meek, V. (2007). Qualitative assignments to enhance online learning. *International Journal of Instructional Technology and Distance Learning, 4*(2), 49–54. Retrieved from http://www.itdl.org/journal/feb_07/Feb_07.pdf

Brookfield, S. D., & Preskill, S. (2005). *Discussions as a way of teaching* (2nd ed.). San Francisco, CA: Jossey-Bass.

Brown, P. C., Roediger, H. L., & McDaniel, M. A. (2014). *Make it stick: The science of successful learning*. Boston, MA: Harvard University Press.

Carnegie Mellon University. (2015). Principles of learning. Retrieved from https://www.cmu.edu/teaching/principles/learning.html

Chickering, A. W., & Gamson, Z. F. (1987). Seven principles for good practice in undergraduate education. Retrieved from http://www.lonestar.edu/multimedia/sevenprinciples.pdf

Fink, L. D. (2013). *Creating significant learning experiences: An integrated approach to designing college courses* (2nd ed.). San Francisco, CA: Jossey-Bass.

Institute of Medicine. (2003). *Health professions education: A bridge to quality*. Washington, DC: National Academies Press.

Knowles, M. (1984). *The adult learner: A neglected species*. Houston, TX: Gulf Publishing.

National Academy of Sciences. (2015). *Reaching students: What research says about effective instruction in undergraduate science and engineering.* Washington, DC: National Academies Press.

Quality and Safety Education for Nurses Institute. (2017). QSEN competencies. Retrieved from http://qsen.org/competencies

Szurmak, J., & Thuna, M. (2013). *Tell me a story: The use of narrative as a tool for instruction.* Conference of the Association of College and Research Libraries, April 10–13, Indianapolis, IN. Retrieved from http://www.ala.org/acrl/acrl/conferences/2013/papers

VARK Learn. (2017). The VARK modalities. Retrieved from http://vark-learn.com/introduction-to-vark/the-vark-modalities/

Walvoord, B. E., & Anderson, V. J. (2009). *Effective grading: A tool for learning and assessment in college.* San Francisco, CA: Jossey-Bass.

CHAPTER 9

Engaging the Learner With Technologies for Feedback, Debriefing, and Evaluation

Gain perspective on the technological options for providing feedback and evaluating student achievement.

BEGINNING REFLECTION

1. What experiences have you had giving feedback to students?
2. With what evaluation techniques are you most familiar and comfortable?
3. How do you use debriefing to help students learn?
4. How can technology promote reasonable and effective evaluations?

Overheard: *Why don't we have a rubric for this assignment?*

The public needs to have confidence that students and graduates in the health professions are safe practitioners. This chapter discusses the use of a variety of technologies to provide feedback and evaluate students. Technology and evaluation are a good match, with technology providing many flexible options for assessment, evaluation, and feedback. Technology can help faculty be fair and consistent. Evaluation is an essential part of the planning process for both courses and assignments. Effective grading involves matching assignments with learning goals. Broad principles of good evaluation developed by the American Association for Higher Education Assessment Forum (Hutchings, Ewell, & Banta, 2012) provide background for this discussion.

Learning management systems and automated response systems (clickers), for example, often provide opportunities for instant testing with immediate feedback that can promote learning. In this chapter, the concepts of feedback and evaluation are considered broadly as learning tools. Evaluation can be both simple and complex. The expectation is to compare student performance with expected outcomes, but the reality is that numerous factors can interfere with that comparison. Although a focus on grades is an inherent part of the educational system and can be a powerful student motivator, a focus only on grades is less likely to encourage a mindset for lifelong learning. Helping students and student groups gain a vision for success is more likely to encourage students toward lifelong learning.

Teaching, learning, and evaluation concepts create a cyclic process and build on one another. Building on assessed needs, new content is typically presented for learning. Students are subsequently evaluated to determine the extent to which goals/objectives for the acquisition of new content were met. The most effective evaluation then becomes a teaching tool to help students with additional learning or to reinforce what has already been learned. Feedback is the process by which students gain information about their performance on the evaluation measures. In addition, evaluation in nursing education is best considered as part of a systematic approach that integrates evaluation across classroom, clinical laboratory, and clinical experiences. Theory application is tested in the classroom; safety competencies are checked off in the learning laboratory; application with patients is gained in the clinical setting.

Why is this topic essential in a book about teaching with technology? First, the explosion of new technologies offers continuously new ways to assess and evaluate students and to provide feedback, so faculty need to know the options and make considered decisions about which to use. Faculty must also be cognizant of the sensitive nature of feedback, especially in a technology-rich world. Sometimes the feedback students must be given is not positive, and faculty need to choose the best and most responsible mechanisms by which to relay this information. As faculty, we must remember that many technological methods, although fast and accessible, are impersonal at best (recall Shea's [1994] classic rules of netiquette). As a result, certain technologies make it harder for faculty to soften negative feedback or determine how students are interpreting and responding to that feedback. More scholarship is still needed for establishing best practices on providing feedback through text-based media.

EVALUATION AND ITS RELATIONSHIP TO TEACHING

Evaluation plays a central role in education. There are a number of related terms, such as assessment and feedback. There are also different types of evaluation, including formative and summative, and norm referenced and criterion referenced. Assessment itself plays an important role in the learning process and remediation activities.

Related Terms: Assessment, Feedback, and Evaluation

Several related terms—assessment, feedback, and evaluation—are often confused or used without regard for their subtle differences. Assessment is the process used to "gather, summarize, interpret, and use data to decide a direction for action (Bastable, 2008, pp. 559-560). Feedback builds on assessment. Feedback has been described as information communicated to students that is based on an assessment and that helps the student reflect and work further with the information provided. This includes reflecting on and creating self-knowledge relevant to course learning and then setting further learning goals (Bonnel, Ludwig, & Smith, 2007). Feedback is usually most effective when it is as timely and objective as possible.

Building on both assessment and feedback, evaluation is the process used to "gather, summarize, interpret, and use data to determine the extent to which an action was successful" (Bastable, 2008, p. 560). Although assessment-based feedback provides direction for actions, evaluation implies a final judgment about the success of actions. Because of this fundamental difference, assessment and feedback are commonly conducted early in the semester and continue in an ongoing fashion throughout the teaching and learning process (to guide further teaching and learning). Evaluation is often conducted later in the semester or process (to establish goal/objective achievement). Evaluation frequently occurs through formal grades but can also occur through ongoing informal mechanisms.

Formative and Summative Evaluation

The process of evaluation is further defined as formative or summative. Formative evaluation is similar to feedback in general and is part of the ongoing learning process. Formative evaluation is conducted during the teaching and learning process to help identify strengths and weaknesses and further guide learning activities. Therefore, formative evaluation and assessment are very similar in nature and may, at times, overlap. Periodic formative evaluations help shape students into proficient nurses. Summative evaluation, on the other hand, implies a final summary of learning and reflects the more conventional view of evaluation that occurs at the end of the teaching and learning process to determine whether objectives/goals were met and to what extent they were met. The evaluation determines whether students have met the criteria of being proficient nurses. Summative evaluation has been described as elevating assessment to the level of making judgments about the quality of students' performance (Billings & Halstead, 2015).

Norm Referenced and Criteria Referenced

Another perspective divides evaluation into norm referenced and criterion referenced. Norm-referenced evaluation compares any given learner with other students or groups of students (either a standardized group or the student's fellow classmates), whereas criterion-referenced evaluation compares the learner with an objective set of criteria. Usually, in norm-referenced evaluations, faculty seek a predetermined distribution of grades that fits a bell curve, with a few students getting very high and very low grades and most earning average grades. In contrast, criterion-referenced evaluation relates to meeting a criterion and does not generally have a predetermined grade distribution. In fact, if all students meet the set of criteria, then all students pass the evaluation; if no students meet the set criteria, then no one passes.

Assessment and Learning

Technology provides multiple opportunities for enhancing assessment of student learning and for providing feedback to students. Assessment can be completed before starting to teach (e.g., lesson, course, laboratory procedure) to see what knowledge students bring with them to the teaching situation. Ongoing assessments, or formative evaluations, may be conducted to determine students' learning to date, identify problems, and help guide the teaching process.

At the beginning of a course or individual class, students can be assessed for their current knowledge level. This assessment may consist of a multiple-choice test in which the testing closes after just 5 or 10 minutes (faculty determined), or it may consist of small group discussion based on the day's required readings. Both options could also be used to conduct formative evaluation as the semester proceeds, or an informal, low-stakes writing exercise during class might provide formative feedback. Summative evaluation may consist of a timed, open-book examination that occurs synchronously for all students, or it may consist of a more formal, high-stakes writing assignment or a formal presentation transmitted to the entire class via video technology.

Hence, we use formative evaluation to help identify students' areas of strength and weakness and to guide their continued learning. We use summative evaluation to determine how much learning has occurred and whether the learning goals were met. Under the best of circumstances, this evaluation then becomes a teaching tool from which students further cement their learning of content and skills. It is easy to forget that the very testing process used for evaluation can itself be a teaching and learning experience. Research suggests that the content-retrieval process required for testing (e.g., multiple-choice or short-answer test) may enhance learning more than simply studying (Weimer, 2015). This insight provides opportunities for combining traditional evaluation methods with new technologies that promote student learning.

Assessment and Remediation

Diverse learning needs and learning styles bring challenges to all classrooms, with the potential need for remediation in selected areas. Remediation, considered a remedy or attempt to improve limited skills, allows students an opportunity to correct errors or deficiencies in needed knowledge. For example, a number of educational testing companies, such as Assessment Technologies Institute (ATI), Health Education Systems, Incorporated (HESI), and Kaplan, offer an array of standardized assessments. Many are based on the concept that students must assess their current knowledge base to identify their achievement to date and then also gain a focused study plan that they can adapt to their own unique knowledge deficits, learning style, and needs. Such standardized assessments offer review, practice, and guidance in weak areas. Remediation is consistent with goal setting and contracting for improved skill sets. As a part of formative evaluation, students can then enhance their abilities to do well on subsequent summative evaluations.

THE MANY FORMS OF FEEDBACK

Feedback is the general term for providing students information about their performance, and technology helps with this process, whether the goal is assessment, formative evaluation, summative evaluation, or remediation. Technology provides many options (with more being discovered every day), often with advantages in efficiency and effectiveness over more traditional evaluation methods. Online quizzes, for example, provide opportunities for multiple reviews. High-fidelity simulations provide technological options in a safe environment in which students can learn new skills (which were formerly learned on real patients).

Also, technologies tend to provide hands-on experience that fit the theoretical principles of active learning discussed in Chapter 3. Technological options also provide a means for ensuring that all students have the same required experiences. For example, if all students in an obstetrics course need to demonstrate the competency of assisting with the delivery of a baby, they all can meet this requirement using simulation; if all students in a critical care course need to provide cardiopulmonary resuscitation (CPR), now they all can. Sample options for using technology in self-assessment/reflection, peer evaluation, rubrics, and debriefing follow.

Self-Assessment and Student Reflection

Although faculty have often been the major source of feedback, there is great value in feedback received from one's own experience and that of peers. Self-assessment based on self-reflection serves many purposes, but among the most important is that it establishes students' role in and responsibility for their own learning. As students assess their own learning gains or deficits, learning that has already occurred can be strengthened or extended as students identify areas for continued growth and learning.

Honest self-reflection can prepare students to be open to feedback from others and to integrate that feedback into their own, self-directed learning. Self-assessment becomes self-evaluation when students judge their performance in comparison with objective criteria. Where there are gaps, self-assessment can help set the path for further learning. Self-assessment provides faculty insight into students' thinking (Driscoll & Wood, 2007). Developing the ability to self-assess is also essential for future professional growth and lifelong learning (Fink, 2013).

In addition to more traditional student evaluation methods, student self-assessment is a common approach for assessing and documenting student learning. Students can be asked in all courses, for example, to complete precourse and postcourse self-assessments against course objectives. In addition to promoting student engagement in the course, this strategy also provides faculty information about student perspectives on status and performance and helps faculty provide better student feedback. An evidence-based review abstract is shared in Exhibit 9.1. This systematic review provides faculty direction for developing reflective assignments for students' clinical activities.

EXHIBIT 9.1

EVIDENCE-BASED REVIEW ABSTRACT: REFLECTIVE JOURNALING

Compiled by: Janet Reagor, PhD, RN

The following summary provides a graduate student's experience of synthesizing literature for her work on reflective journaling.

THE CHALLENGE

Reflective writing is useful in developing critical thinking skills, assisting in coping with stressful situations, and facilitating personal and professional growth. For reflective writing to be effective, the technique must be valued by the individual. Reflective writing is a skill that is developed with practice. By encouraging students to learn and develop reflective writing skills, they will, it is hoped, continue to use this strategy after graduation, when it may have an impact on their own growth and satisfaction in the role of the professional nurse and have a positive impact on patient outcomes.

SYNTHESIS/INTERPRETATION OF CURRENT LITERATURE

Journals are a widely accepted method of encouraging students to reflect on both their successes and less-than-perfect performances during their clinical experiences. Journals encourage students to look beyond the facts of the incident, to explore the implications of the event, to understand how alternative actions would have affected the event, and how they reacted to the event.

A systematic review of the literature supports the use of reflection in clinical journals, with opinions varying as to the role of grading journal entries. Many authors felt that grading the journal entries forced students to write not for their own benefit, but for pleasing the instructor. Although some authors recommended the use of guided questions to facilitate student writing, other authors felt that this would stifle student creativity. All authors recommended that if journals are graded, they should be evaluated only on the use of the reflective process and not on the activities associated with the recorded incident. Several rubrics for evaluating the reflective process are available, varying widely in length, depth, and descriptors.

ONGOING ISSUES FOR STUDY

Several grading rubrics were found in the literature, but most were quite lengthy and would be time consuming for clinical instructors to use for grading. The ideal grading rubric should be short and clearly outline the process to be followed when writing the clinical journal. If, as many authors advocated, the journals are not graded, then further study on how to encourage students to be involved in the process of reflective journaling is needed.

Peer Evaluation

Peer evaluation is an important tool by which students learn skills for the future. It is an important part of students' roles on clinical teams. Benefits of peer evaluation include learning opportunities and exchange by sharing feedback with others. Criteria to promote fair peer evaluation include clear standards and guides and explanation of the professional role of the evaluator. Given the proper guidance, students can use peer evaluation to provide meaningful feedback. Whether peers are fellow students or fellow clinical staff, it is critical that they be given clear evaluation guidelines and that they evaluate only content or skills that they are prepared to evaluate. Thus, effective orientation to this skill is important. Orientation includes not only what students will be doing, but also why they will be doing it. Peer evaluation promotes the concept of professional responsibility, and it helps develop the collaborative skills required to work effectively in teams. Peer feedback is also a needed lifelong skill.

As with all forms of evaluation, the primary challenge to effective self-assessment and peer evaluation is the potential for bias. The essential element is honesty, and, when honesty is present, personal and peer feedback are helpful to both students and faculty. Sometimes students may be too hard on themselves or too easy on their peers (although the opposite can also be true).

Rubrics

Rubrics are developed to grade an assignment (either formative or summative), as well as to provide students guidance in assignment completion. These are good evaluation tools for many reasons. A rubric is an explicit summary, often in list form, of essential criteria for a project, with rating potential for each criterion. Faculty use of rubrics can promote timely, detailed feedback responses, encourage critical thinking, and facilitate student–faculty communication (Stevens & Levi, 2005). They have the benefit of providing more detailed information than a specific letter grade alone.

Rubrics can vary from simple to complex. A simple rubric for a writing assignment, for example, might include basic criteria for content and organization. Good rubrics help students focus on what is important to learn rather than treating all facts as equally important. Rubrics provide both a learning tool and an evaluation tool. They are also beneficial for self-assessment and student peer review. Rubrics provide a guide for learning and project development for students and thus serve as tools for teaching self-directed learning. Providing rubrics at the initiation of an assignment gives students better direction on assignment expectations. Faculty can find that these tools make grading easier and more consistent. Good rubrics are more than just a checklist. Quality Matters (2017) provides excellent resources for rubric development and use.

Debriefing as a Type of Feedback

Debriefing also provides an opportunity for feedback. Debriefing after a clinical or simulated experience, for example, provides (often in a group setting) the opportunity to assess what happened, compare this to accepted criteria, and consider what worked or did not work. The National League for Nursing (NLN, 2016) provides a guide for helping teach students to think through such experiences. Faculty are directed to help students tell the patient's story, guide their thinking about the situation, and integrate learning into their practice. Ask students questions about the context (what were your concerns about this patient, and how did you feel taking care of him?), content (what were your thoughts during the experience, and what have you previously learned that influenced your actions?), and course (what would your next actions be, and what would you do differently next time?). An important component of debriefing is asking students to engage in further goal setting or to address what learning is still needed. Although debriefing is becoming a fairly common source of feedback, there is still a lot to learn about best debriefing practices. Neill and Wotton (2011) conducted a review of the debriefing literature in nursing and, based on seven articles from the United States and two from Australia, found wide variation in current practices and a lot of gaps in the research.

SELECTED TECHNOLOGIES AND EVALUATION AND FEEDBACK

A growing number of technological advances facilitate evaluation and learning processes. Selected items discussed here include clickers, learning management systems, standardized computer testing, simulation, and clinical competencies.

Classroom Response Systems (Clickers)

Clickers consist of both classroom hardware and software that connect students, faculty, and audiovisual media. Students have small handheld devices that enable them to express their answers or views anonymously to other students in the classroom in aggregate form. The anonymous feature allows all students to participate, whether in a large class that would otherwise prohibit participation of all students or in a smaller class with students reluctant to express their individual views. Some automated-response programs offer faculty the ability to track individual student responses.

Clickers have the added benefit of providing immediate feedback to students and faculty, so they can identify areas for additional time and attention. Clickers can be used at the beginning of class as a preassessment or used for assessment of students' understanding of assigned readings. They can be used throughout a class period to provide ongoing feedback for students and faculty. Clickers can also be used as an evaluation technique at the end of a class period, with the advantage of providing virtually instantaneous feedback.

Learning Management Systems

Whether in a face-to-face course or an online course, computer-based classroom management systems are fast becoming the norm. Although these systems provide a mechanism by which to organize course content (and computer links) and make it available to students at their convenience, they also provide multiple opportunities for teaching, learning, and evaluation (hence learning, rather than classroom, management systems). These systems provide a mechanism by which students can take examinations (timed or not) and participate in online discussions (both synchronous and asynchronous). Grades can be posted so that students have access to their ongoing grade status. Although testing is just one aspect of evaluation, it is an important one because of its often high-stakes nature. If testing is the evaluation tool used, test questions need to be aligned with course goals (Driscoll & Wood, 2007; Fink, 2013). For example, if the lesson goal is critical thinking and just memorized information is tested, the test is not well aligned with teaching and learning goals.

Learning management systems provide item analysis opportunities to review test item performance. They provide opportunities to seek reliability and validity in the objective tests the faculty implement. Many technologies are now available to promote easy review with an item analysis. Additional detail can often be gained from add-on programs. Technology provides the opportunity to make testing more reliable and valid, which, in a high-stakes testing situation, helps ensure fair testing. Item analysis becomes much easier with tools provided by learning management systems or added packages to review computer-based testing. More details concerning learning management systems is found in Chapter 11.

Standardized Computer Testing

Testing can also be used as a tool for instruction. Whether for actual testing situations or practice testing, computerized testing programs provide further learning opportunities. As mentioned earlier, online testing programs such as ATI, HESI, and Kaplan provide the opportunity for students to participate in self-directed learning assessments. These practice tests can help prepare students for safe, knowledgeable practice as outlined by national boards.

This approach is different from testing in which students earn a grade but do not clearly understand the areas where they are not performing well. Automated practice tests can provide students immediate feedback on individual answers. Students gain benchmarks in matching their scores to others. If properly oriented, students can benefit from knowing where their weaknesses are and what learning areas they need to focus on. In addition, students gain individualized learning plans with areas of study outlined.

Simulations

High-fidelity patient simulation (HFPS) provides multiple options for assessing, evaluating, and remediating content. For example, faculty might teach and/or assess current student knowledge by walking students through a scenario as it unfolds step by step. This process helps students integrate information and witness the faculty's rationale for decisions, as well as observe the HFPS patient's response to the actions taken. This approach might be appropriate for very new or very complicated content. Formative evaluation might consist of placing students in a scenario and letting it unfold naturally, according to the decisions (appropriate or not) that the students make and implement. For example, place students in a scenario where the HFPS patient unexpectedly codes and watch how the scenario unfolds. The use of rubrics for the experience would provide students rapid feedback on the quality of their performance, and that same rubric could be used for the final, summative evaluation at semester's end.

The debriefing experience, particularly during the semester as formative evaluation, is an excellent opportunity for students to apply learned content, think through rationales on which to base their actions, and clarify questions. It also enables students to evaluate their own critical thinking skills by comparing their rationale to that of other students and faculty. The NLN (2017) Center for Innovation in Simulation and Technology provides rich resources in the form of educational webinars and simulation scenarios to support and advance the use of technology across curricula. Additional content on simulation is also presented in Chapter 12.

Clinical Competencies

Clinical evaluation is multifaceted and often includes summative evaluation related to competencies. Technology is particularly useful in evaluating competencies with resources such as computer programs, learning laboratories, and HFPS. Further discussion of clinical evaluation with technology is included in Chapters 12 and 14.

Emerging technologies provide clinical experiences in a safe and controlled environment in which faculty can direct and control students' experiences. They also represent a fairly flexible teaching format that provides access to multiple students at their own convenience. Because of these features, technology provides a mechanism by which to address the Quality and Safety Education for Nurses Institute (QSEN, 2017) and Interprofessional Education Collaborative (IPEC, 2016) clinical competencies. For example, the call for an emphasis on interprofessional education is hard to accomplish when medical schools, nursing schools, and pharmacy schools all operate on very different schedules (for both didactic and clinical experiences). However, a virtual hospital created in Second Life can provide the mechanism by which all three professions can work together, asynchronously if needed, so that incompatible schedules do not preclude the opportunity to work, learn, and practice concepts of interprofessional teamwork together. Potential for competency evaluation also exists via these venues.

TRIANGLE OF INTEGRATED LEARNING FOR TEACHING WITH TECHNOLOGIES

The concept of integrated or deep learning achievement with technologies is central to this text. The content presented in this chapter falls soundly in the Integrated Learning Triangle for Teaching With Technologies; a major component in that triangle includes assessment, feedback, and evaluation. As discussed, technology provides many opportunities to help students achieve this integrated learning.

SUMMARY

Technology provides a wide variety of choices for providing student assessment, evaluation, and feedback. Optimizing various opportunities for feedback via assignment design creates multiple learning opportunities. Technologies such as online learning management systems create effective and efficient mechanisms for faculty use, as well as student learning opportunities. Human simulators are another example of technology that can be used to evaluate students' competencies and provide feedback. Technology provides both formative and summative evaluation opportunities to help guide student learning and progress toward independent clinical practice, interprofessional teamwork, and lifelong learning.

ENDING REFLECTIONS FOR YOUR LEARNING NOTEBOOK

1. What is the most important content that you learned in this chapter?
2. What are your plans for using the information provided in this chapter in your future teaching endeavors?
3. What are your further learning goals?

GUIDELINES FOR TEACHING AND LEARNING WITH TECHNOLOGIES

Quick Teaching Tips

1. Beginning assessments—whether at the beginning of a semester or the start of an individual class day—let both you and students know what knowledge gaps exist and identify what needs to be learned.
2. Use multiple sources for evaluation, and check between the sources for consistency; if consistency is lacking, consider possible explanations and their implications for student learning.
3. Always find something positive to say about student performance.

Questions for Further Reflection

1. Can all feedback be considered good feedback? What are some considerations related to this question?
2. What strategies do you use to provide formative feedback to students?
3. What strategies do you use to challenge students to self-reflect and set further learning goals? How do these strategies contribute to active learning and critical thinking?
4. What are the benefits and limitations of various technological options for evaluation?

5. Will the use of technological options such as simulation and gaming improve student learning in a meaningful way?
6. What information will you use to make a decision (in the Triangle of Integrated Learning for Teaching With Technologies) regarding which technology to use?
7. What is meant by high- and low-stake evaluation? What tools are used by other fields to measure and improve individual competency? Can those tools be applied to nursing?
8. What are benefits of competency-based education and training for individuals, for agencies, and for society?

Learning Activity: Exploring Different Evaluation Options and their Application to Teaching and Learning Situations

You are teaching a course in which students are presenting group projects on a semester-long community teaching activity. Your syllabus says the presentation evaluation will consist of self-evaluation, peer evaluation, and faculty evaluation.

1. What type of evaluation criteria or rubric will you expect each of these three rating groups to use?
2. If using a rubric, will each rating group (self, peer, and faculty) use the same rubric criteria? Whether you chose the same or different rubric criteria for each group, explain your rationale.

A year later, you are teaching the same course. In trying to improve students' grades this year, you decide to add a formative project evaluation at mid-semester so that students get feedback as they work on the projects/presentations.

1. Will criteria you use for the mid-semester evaluation be the same or different from the evaluation criteria you use at the end of the semester? Explain the rationale for your decision.

Online Resources for Further Learning

■ Carnegie Mellon, Teaching with Clickers. This site holds links to a variety of topics, including assessment and clickers. www.cmu.edu/teaching/index.html
■ University of Virginia, Teaching Resource Center. This site contains links to numerous teaching resources, including "course evaluations" and "grading." trc.virginia.edu/Publications/Teaching_Concerns/TC_Topic.htm
■ University of Wisconsin–Madison, National Institute for Science Education, Field-tests Learning Assessment Guide (FLAG). This site offers a variety of resources, including classroom assessment techniques, through which you can find links to concept mapping and rubrics, among others. archive.wceruw.org/cl1/flag/cat/cat.htm

REFERENCES

Bastable, S. B. (2017). *Nurse as educator: Principles of teaching and learning for nursing practice.* Sudbury, MA: Jones & Bartlett.

Billings, D. M., & Halstead, J. A. (2015). *Teaching in nursing: A guide for faculty* (5th ed.). St. Louis, MO: Saunders Elsevier.

Bonnel, W., Ludwig, C., & Smith, J. (2007). Providing feedback in online courses: What do students want? How do we do that? *Annual Review of Nursing Education, 6,* 205–221.

Driscoll, A., & Wood, S. (2007). *Developing outcomes-based assessment for learner-centered education: A faculty introduction.* Sterling, VA: Stylus.

Fink, L. D. (2013). *Creating significant learning experiences: An integrated approach to designing college courses.* San Francisco, CA: Jossey-Bass.

Hutchings, P., Ewell, P., & Banta, T. (2012). AAHE Principles of good practice: Aging nicely. Retrieved from http://learningoutcomesassessment.org/PrinciplesofAssessment.html#AAHE

Interprofessional Education Collaborative. (2016). *Core competencies for interprofessional collaborative practice: 2016 update.* Washington, DC: Author.

National League for Nursing. (2016). Critical conversations: The NLN guide for teaching thinking. Retrieved from http://www.nln.org/search?query=critical%20conversations

National League for Nursing. (2017). NLN Center for Innovation in Simulation and Technology. Retrieved from http://www.nln.org/centers-for-nursing-education/nln-center-for-innovation-in-simulation-and-technology2

Neill, M. A., & Wotton, K. (2011). High-fidelity simulation debriefing in nursing education: A literature review. Retrieved from http://www.nursingsimulation.org/article/S1876-1399(11)00026-0/pdf

Quality and Safety Education for Nurses Institute. (2017). QSEN competencies. Retrieved from http://qsen.org/competencies

Quality Matters. (2017). The quality matters rubric. Retrieved from https://www.qualitymatters.org/qa-resources/rubric-standards

Shea, V. (1994). *Netiquette.* San Francisco, CA: Albion Books.

Stevens, D., & Levi, A. (2005). *Introduction to rubrics: An assessment tool to save grading time, convey effective feedback, and promote student learning.* Sterling VA: Stylus.

Weimer, M. (2015). Testing that promotes learning. Retrieved from https://tomprof.stanford.edu/posting/1593

Diverse Clinical Practice and Educational Technologies

Online Education: Maximizing the Opportunities for Learning Populations and Systems Care

CHAPTER GOAL

Consider best practices for teaching and learning in an online environment.

BEGINNING REFLECTION

1. What does the concept of online learning mean to you?
2. What are your best experiences teaching in an online environment?
3. What has been your most challenging experience teaching with technology?

Overheard: *How can I teach them if I can't see them?*

Online learning has changed education. Online learning provides the opportunity to bring the world in, connecting beyond the confines of the learning management system. The Internet makes it possible to connect with experts or resources from across the state or worldwide.

Faculty have a baseline in traditional teaching modes but are now facilitating learning in new ways online. Online learning has provided opportunities to reflect on our traditional teaching modes and examine what works and what does not in the online setting. Much has been written about the online classroom because it has led to major changes in all arenas, including nursing education. Online education has presented a major stimulus for reconsidering our pedagogy as healthcare educators.

Both benefits and challenges exist in online education. Although online education benefits include flexibility for students, challenges often exist in engaging learners and making content interactive. Trying to create online the same effect as in a face-to-face classroom typically does not work. For example, just because it is now possible to lecture online does not necessarily mean that particular mode best accomplishes course objectives. This chapter focuses on the pedagogy of online learning rather than learning management systems in courses that meet entirely online without a face-to-face component. This chapter provides an overview of opportunities and strategies for enhancing online courses for health professional students.

WHY WE MEET OUR STUDENTS ONLINE

Learning online provides students advantages in a number of ways. Benefits of access and timeliness to online learning, including ongoing access to course and web resources, geographic flexibility, and time flexibility, are key. The Internet affords a wide variety of learning opportunities that help meet students' diverse learning styles and personal needs. Faculty have more opportunities for interaction with students, compared with scheduled weekly class sessions often held in the classroom. Faculty gain opportunities to receive comments from all students. Often students gain the opportunity to learn from diverse populations and gain access to a wide range of individuals that likely would not happen in one classroom.

Online and self-directed learning are particularly intertwined; online methods promote learner responsibility and preparation for self-directed learning. Fink (2013) points out that learning how to learn is a critical concept. Faculty guide or coach students in learning skills and concepts to prepare for the profession. Students gain opportunities in a structured venue for developing self-directed learning skills. In particular, online learning starts best with good orientations, not only to the course, but also to learning online.

WHAT WE MEAN BY AN ONLINE COURSE

Terms for online education vary and include web-based learning, e-learning, online learning, virtual classes, and others. Palloff and Pratt (2001) note that trying to describe online education, with its rapidity of change, is like trying to describe a fast-moving river. Online learning descriptions are also complicated by the additional concepts of synchronous and asynchronous learning. Synchronous learning describes experiences completed in real time. Asynchronous learning, such as used with online discussion boards, takes place at staggered times. Broad principles can provide direction in dealing with this rapidly moving resource.

Online education, starting primarily as text-based learning, has grown rapidly to encompass a variety of teaching and learning opportunities and approaches. Although online education has been offered with a book and study questions, much is missing if online courses are not expanded to incorporate best practices (see the following discussion of best practices). A major benefit to online education is the broad connections with the world; this link is missed if students are provided just a book and a study guide within the confines of a learning management system. Technology allows online courses to use a variety of features, including interactive assignments such as surveys, discussions, and authentic learning assignments (e.g., online student posters and presentations). Opportunities for applied assignments such as interviews and observations related to clinical learning are also available. These tools take us a long way in expanding on the previously text-based learning.

Particularly in online courses, engaging students to actively do something with the information presented is central in learning. For example, in an online nursing informatics class, reading a book and taking quizzes on content can be one approach. Using that approach, however, students lose many learning opportunities if they do not also engage in applied assignments and online discussions within the learning community. The latter approach helps students to further consider how the information applies in their own or future clinical settings.

BEST PRACTICES IN ONLINE TEACHING, SELECTED MODELS

What is the pedagogy behind the technology for online education? Best educational practices consistent with adult education theory are considered guides. Online education was evaluated by Chickering and Ehrman's (1996) classic reference on best practices as applied to online education. Evidence-supported learning practices described by Carnegie Mellon University (2015) are consistent with active learning. Based on best practices, optimal learning is more likely to occur if faculty do more than just choose a textbook and place a study guide online. Interactive courses help engage students in learning content.

Teaching and learning online should implement practices that contribute to effective, efficient, and satisfying experiences. Individual students learn within a community facilitated by the faculty (Boettcher, 2011; Hanover Research Council, 2009). Suggested best practices for teaching online include incorporating:

Presence and Caring:
- Be present in the course (communicates caring, interaction, and cohesion).
- Create a supportive course community (facilitates peer and instructor coaching with problem solving).
Diverse approaches that include clear expectations:
- Share clear expectations (includes student, course, and instructor).

- Integrate a variety of individual and group learning activities (addresses diverse learning needs).
- Assemble synchronous and asynchronous assignments (engages learners in collaborative and reflective learning).
- Deploy applications that encourage learners to incorporate current events (encourages students to integrate the world of Internet resources).
- Interlink course core concepts with personalized learning (guides students to create concept awareness with intellectual acquisition).

Feedback and questioning throughout:

- Complete early, periodic, and ongoing course evaluations (connects with students in real time to increase course satisfaction and learning);
- Integrate discussion posts that invite questions and responses (encourages critical thinking and community building);
- Plan for course closure (create opportunities for knowledge integration with reflection).

Interactive courses help engage students in learning content. Sample websites that support best practices in online education are listed in Exhibit 10.1.

Using best practices in teaching and learning as guides, the following concepts are discussed as tools for promoting successful online education: concepts of course design, facilitating applied active learning, and feedback to students. In addition, it is important to consider generational differences. As Faculty Champion Jan Foecke explained, there are important concepts to consider within, between, and respective to student generations that will impact teaching and learning results. She describes examples such as detailed instructions, depth and frequency of announcements, technology application requirements, group work, facilitating peer review, and downplaying differences among learners (see Exhibit 10.2).

EXHIBIT 10.1

WEBSITES THAT SUPPORT BEST PRACTICES

Websites that support best practices in teaching and learning online education include:

- The Teaching, Learning, and Technology (TLT) Group. A group providing faculty support in using changing technologies: www.tltgroup.org
- Walker Center for Teaching and Learning. A resource that implements Chickering and Gamson's *Seven Principles for Good Practice in Undergraduate Education* for faculty practice and strategy applications: www.utc.edu/walker-center-teaching-learning/teaching-resources/7-principles.php
- Designing for Learning. A resource that highlights ten best practices for teaching online: www.designingforlearning.info/services/writing/ecoach/tenbest.html

EXHIBIT 10.2

TIPS FROM FACULTY CHAMPIONS: BETTER UNDERSTANDING GENERATIONS ONLINE Q&A

Jan Foecke, PhD, MS, RN, ONC

1. ***What is your current position like, relevant to teaching with diverse generations online?*** I currently teach a foundational course in a graduate nursing school that includes learners from generation X, Millennial generation, and i-Generation. I also facilitate CNE programs for all faculty members in our school of nursing. The CNE presenters are generally from the Baby Boomer, Generation X, and Millennial generations, and the faculty learners are from four generations: Silent, Baby Boomer, Generation X, and Millennials. The presentations occur in webinar format and are recorded with required online Blackboard components for faculty learners (e.g., access recorded program, handout, attendance verification, post-test, and evaluation).

2. ***What ways do you see your faculty or students benefiting from a better understanding of diverse generations?*** My 2017 doctoral dissertation was specific to examining generational theory to enhance online CNE. Both the literature review and my qualitative research interviews yielded evidence to support many varied generational preferences for learning online in CNE.

3. ***What are some of the major differences you find with diverse student generations online?*** *What are key points faculty would need to better understand related to teaching and learning needs of these diverse groups?* Some major differences of the diverse learner generations online include extent of self-directedness; degree of comfort with technology; preferred methods of learning; desire for and approach to individual assignments versus team-oriented assignments; desired frequency of feedback; and completion of life lessons that influence the quality of scholarly work. There are some key ideas that may be useful toward better understanding of teaching and learning needs of the diverse learner generations, such as providing detailed instructions and frequent reminders to multigenerational learners because of different levels of self-directedness; posting detailed instructions/tutorials about the use of the technology associated with an online course due to technological skill; incorporating multiple methods of instruction and learning; and assigning various generational members to work groups to facilitate sharing of strengths and downplay differences among learners. In general, Millennials and iGeneration learners (iGens) prefer frequent and immediate feedback about their performances and often need extra feedback with further instructions to best understand meeting the criteria of an assignment.

4. ***Should different teaching and learning styles be considered in different generations?*** *How do you manage to keep a student-focused learning approach with diverse generations?* Yes, different teaching and learning styles should be considered for different generations. The findings gathered from qualitative interviews of multigenerational nurses yielded strong and varied recommendations for incorporation into online learning that better meets the learning needs of individual generations. Keeping in mind that every member of a generation is not exactly like the next member of the same generation helps to maintain a learner-focused approach to education. In addition, using formative evaluations while encouraging learners to be accountable and responsible to share their needs with faculty facilitates a learner-focused approach.

(continued)

5. ***What are select facilitators for addressing diverse generational learning needs into your online nursing education courses/programs?*** Providing specific criteria for learners to meet when developing individual bios is useful to better recognize the likely generation of each learner. Bios assist in understanding information such as levels of experience and intended career goals, as well as professional characteristics for assigning diverse learners to groups for team projects. Providing various types of assignments while incorporating selectable options within the assignments is geared toward meeting a higher volume of the diverse learning needs of a multigenerational group. A key point is to offer detailed individual feedback to each learner about assignments, as well as more generic feedback to all learners throughout a course.

6. ***What are select challenges of addressing diverse generational learning needs into your online nursing education courses/programs?*** One challenge to addressing diverse generational learning needs is the time and effort required to create selectable options from which learners can choose to better meet their generational learning needs and preference. Partnering with a learning technology specialist can be very beneficial when creating those options. Maintaining current and developing new technological skills can be challenging, but is necessary, for faculty to educate multigenerational learners, especially Millennials and iGens. In addition, incorporating the use of social media into online courses can be challenging because of confidentiality requirements of higher education.

7. ***What is a favorite assignment/recommendation for a student-focused learning approach? How do you manage to stay creative with your approaches?*** Multigenerational learners have varied experience levels with writing professional papers. In addition to giving feedback on individual papers, I post Writing Tips for Future Professional Papers in the course announcements after all papers have been graded for each assignment. The Writing Tips include recommendations related to common themes identified throughout grading of all learner papers and are organized according to title page, body, and reference page. I often gain creative ideas when addressing learner questions in emails, by reading comments in course discussion forums by reviewing other online courses, and by reading articles about online approaches to learning.

8. ***What tips or advice would you like to share with new faculty teaching online with diverse generations?*** First, identify your own generational biases. In other words, evaluate your beliefs in comparison with those learners that are within your generation and those from other generations. Other faculty tips include educating yourself about the various learning preferences of learners from each generation to provide methods/tools to better meet diverse learning preferences and needs; involve varied learners and professionals in developing course activities; educate learners about some of the learning preferences from the different generations; and mix up group membership so that there are different generations represented in each group.

CNE, continuing nursing education.

CONCEPTS OF DESIGN IN ONLINE COURSES

Design and lesson planning concepts intertwine. Weimer (2013) described faculty as designers who create challenging assignments and then provide the environment for success. Lesson plan principles guide the design phase as we move from classroom to online venues (our classroom teaching and learning experiences help us think about what we want to accomplish). Guided by the Integrated Learning Triangle for Teaching With Technologies (Exhibit 1.3), we use approaches similar to lesson plans but typically organize materials into

EXHIBIT 10.3

ONLINE TEACHING STRATEGIES TO BUILD THE LEARNING COMMUNITY

Designing courses that develop a robust online learning community can include a "big picture" calendar approach to a course. Attending to beginnings, middles, and endings in online course design promotes efficient course facilitation. Sample approaches to using concepts of beginnings, middles, and ending for organizing include the following:

BEGINNINGS: USING BEST PRACTICES TO SET THE STAGE FOR LEARNING

- Gain knowledge of the learners.
- Orient learners to the class and to the technologies.
- Create class set.

MIDDLES/TRANSITIONS: TECHNOLOGIES, AND FACILITATING APPLIED/AUTHENTIC LEARNING

- Make learning active and authentic to engage the learning community.
- Create meaningful assignments.
- Use our educator repositories (an example is Robert Wood Johnson Foundation's Quality and Safety Education for Nurses Institute).

ENDINGS: TECHNOLOGIES, FEEDBACK, AND DEBRIEFING

- Use feedback and debriefing.
- Use rubrics to promote feedback ease and reliability.
- Use self-reflection and portfolios as opportunities to synthesize authentic learning.
- Create closure.

a modular type electronic format. As discussed in Chapter 4, clear and relevant objectives are critical to online assignment and course design.

As we move courses online or design new courses in an online format, thinking about what needs to be retained from the classroom and what new strategies are needed provides direction for online design. Class organizing plans come in many shapes and sizes, and in almost all cases, they influence classroom accomplishments. Similar in arrangement to more traditional learning modules, good formats include objectives, resources, and activities. Authors cite the importance of integrating and aligning assessment (and feedback) with course learning goals and teaching and learning activities, affirming that appropriate course design can help alleviate later problems in the course. As noted in the Integrated Learning Triangle for Teaching With Technologies (Exhibit 1.3), learning objectives, learning activities, and feedback and evaluation make up the points of the triangle, providing direction for course design.

Focusing on the assignments and relevant feedback that lead to course outcomes guides students in mastering content. One approach is to consider the big picture of the online course around course phases. Focusing on course phases during the design phase (calendar view of the course) maintains the teaching and learning flow from beginning to end (see Exhibit 10.3). These concepts provide direction for integrating technology and facilitating student learning in creating assignments that begin the course, move it along, and then bring closure.

When using best practices to facilitate learning with a "calendar" view of the course, "beginnings" acknowledge that learning communities are groups of people engaged in common learning goals. Strategies such as those noted in Exhibit 10.2 help diverse generations come together to learn with and about technologies. Addressing course "middles" recognizes that technology can bring the world to students. As faculty consider applications and authentic learning that can be a part of online learning, we help add high touch to a high-technology world. Specific to course endings, faculty have a coaching role in providing student feedback, as well as debriefing intense learning experiences. Feedback and debriefing are especially important in online environments, helping deepen and cement student learning.

A variety of approaches help students learn online. Varying types of assignments allow diverse opportunities for interactions with content and help meet diverse learners needs. Varied approaches such as voice, video, and print can be combined to create unique online learning opportunities. Questions can guide course decisions, such as: Do audio or video components enhance or support learning opportunities? What are the advantages and disadvantages of each in helping students learn and use information?

Further questions to stimulate thinking about features to be designed into courses include the following:

- Will you incorporate audio or lecture online such as a podcast or classroom capture?
- Will you incorporate visuals (online videos/other)?
- Will you use applied assignments with interactions? (See next section.)
- Will you use group assignments?
- Will you use quizzes and responses to cases to provide a way to document attainment/mastery of the content?

O'Neil (2014) describes a decision tree for online course development. She also recommends a quality check of course pages, as well as field testing and piloting of online course modules prior to the course start date. Copyright issues when using materials developed by others should also be considered.

FACILITATING APPLIED ACTIVE LEARNING

Applied learning assignments are particularly relevant to enhance content in online learning. Although online education in the past was often text based, readings or written content presentations alone do not provide active support of learning. Active learning involves working with the content in some way, such as applying it to cases or interacting via quizzes or other assignments. Engaging active learning assignments help students use and understand the content.

A focus on student success in online learning is particularly important in online education, in which face-to-face contact is usually missing. Synthesis of research supports that active learning helps students gain and retain learning (National Academy of Sciences, 2015). When students use active learning opportunities online to engage with a topic, they better attend to content. A variety of tools (e.g., cases, website reviews, and authentic assignments), appropriately paired with learning concepts, can promote the integration of information needed to guide students in providing safe, quality patient care.

Cases

Case examples and problem-based learning serve as a type of role play, providing opportunity to visualize and bring to life concepts and processes. Cases involve learner-content interaction that requires critical thinking. The questioning that students bring to case study work and to problem-based learning helps them actively use concepts in preparing for clinical care. The questioning afforded by these methods helps them better put content into context, leading to enhanced clinical judgment and safety in care approaches (Benner, Tanner, & Chesla, 2009). Case study and other inquiry-based methods help students take responsibility for their learning as they identify issues, frame questions, seek resources, and identify care solutions (McKeachie & Svinicki, 2014) for their specialized clinical areas.

Website Reviews

Although faculty have always focused on helping students with acquiring information, information is now so readily available that not only access, but also critique, is important. Weimer (2013) noted the need to discover how best to teach with a world at our fingertips. It can be beneficial to extend courses beyond the confines of the learning management system to capture aspects of the broader world. Helping students use best-evidence Internet resources, as discussed in Chapter 5, also serves as a tool for promoting self-directed and lifelong learning; students graduating as self-directed learners gain further learning opportunities from familiarity with important clinical Internet resources.

Authentic Assignments

Broad categories of interactive, authentic assignments include interview, observation, and document review (Bonnel & Meek, 2007). As discussed in Chapter 8, these tools provide flexibility in teaching to different types of learners and diverse groups. They also provide numerous opportunities for students to learn from each other's experiences. Sample ways students can explore and learn about clinical practice include the following:

- **_Developing applied products._** Applied products can include a project developed by students to demonstrate their learning while meeting a particular need. Incorporating projects into learning plans builds on good educational practices and provides an authentic product for peer and faculty review.

- **Interviews**. Online sharing of interview summaries from mentors or others provides opportunity to compare experiences and their similarities and differences in how things are done. For students, interviews may even serve as access to new settings, providing introductions even to future mentoring opportunities.
- **Document reviews.** Sharing document reviews, such as patient education resources on the Internet, students not only select an issue or problem to share but also review multiple teaching resources on the topic and consider the benefits or problems with each, selecting one as a tool for practice. As students share their work via online discussion groups, all students gain a variety of resources for their own practice.
- **Observations.** Projects specific to observation-type assignments, such as patient education groups or support groups in relevant courses, provide students opportunity to learn about nursing care with places limited only by the geography of the students.

An example of authentic learning in a patient education nursing elective includes an observational assignment as previously noted. In this observation assignment, students observe a group education session and complete a brief report. Students are then asked to share key bullet points specific to the people, the place, and the process involved. As students reflect and share in the online discussion, they gain information from these observations of educational groups in different settings (such as rural and urban), different specialties, and different-sized settings. Instead of learning from only one group observation, a class of 20 students gain group teaching tips from 20 different patient educators. Further description of this course and teaching and learning examples are provided in Exhibit 10.4, with examples from a nursing elective in patient education.

ADDING REFLECTION TO APPLIED LEARNING

Adding reflection to applied learning further cements learning (Fink, 2013). For example, with applied learning projects, students can enhance their learning by reflecting and conversing with others about these experiences. Since students often complete applied learning projects at sites distant from one another, there are benefits to moving their reflections and discussions online. Reflection promotes learning as students synthesize what they have learned and share their learning with others.

Discussion Groups Online

Online discussions often serve as a central focus of an online course, serving as a way for the online learning community to connect and share. Online classes (missing classroom immediacy. as well as verbal and nonverbal prompts) change the context for faculty and student discussions and questioning. Technology brings online discussion opportunities that allow unique ways of

EXHIBIT 10.4

BSN ELECTIVE "PATIENT EDUCATION FOR DIVERSE POPULATIONS," EXAMPLES OF APPLIED LEARNING

The patient education course for nurses completing their BSN provides opportunities for students to reflect on possible future educator roles. The course is designed to develop the health professional's role as patient educator and to promote a skill set to enhance teaching and learning for diverse multicultural patient populations. Students gain experiences assessing the learning needs of a target population and developing educational programs. Participants apply current learning theories and effective teaching strategies to design, implement, and evaluate educational experiences for diverse learners. Technological advances, as well as current and future issues in patient and clinical education, are considered.

Context: RN to BSN population. Active online participation has particular appeal for younger groups who see the Internet as a comfortable place to extend their learning.

Course methods: Based on adult learning theory, the eight-module course integrates active learning and applied assignments. Online content such as Healthy People 2020 and recent IOM reports on patient safety provide easily accessible readings to complement more traditional resources.

Engaging assignments: Students share cultural competence briefings with classmates, gain awareness of health literacy issues and communication tools, assess their practice sites for cultural competence, reflect on patient Internet use and critique websites for their educational potential. They gain a skill set for actively involving patients in their learning, identify new evaluation approaches, and critique interprofessional patient education approaches. An applied project in the form of a teaching plan that students pilot in patient care is included as well.

Process: Assignments are designed with an applied focus, including interviews of an experienced patient educator, observations of a patient education group teaching session, and reviews of online patient teaching resources. The majority of student assignments are then shared in summary format at an online discussion board.

In addition, students review online resources to enhance student cultural competence and patient teaching for diverse populations. A sample assignment is a cultural debriefing provided to student colleagues on an online discussion board. Health-promotion websites, such as Healthy People 2020, that have topic relevance are used for a patient health-promotion teaching session.

Benefits and evaluation: Access to diverse websites and applied learning experiences provide authentic learning that transfers to students' future practice. Websites reviewed are available for students to catalog for future clinical practice. Using active learning strategies gives students practice in becoming more self-directed learners. Student fast-feedback forms, student projects, course evaluations, and student surveys from this RN-to-BSN elective support that students learn educator skills and, in many cases, expand their thinking to consider future faculty roles.

IOM, Institute of Medicine.

bringing diverse groups together. Some tips for interesting, successful discussions include the following:

- Clearly identify faculty roles (and expectations), as well as student roles in participating and processing discussions.
- Provide orientation and clear guidelines as to the discussion purpose and process.
- Provide interesting topics such as those with controversy, including interesting discussion prompts as the discussion progresses.
- Consider strategies for facilitating the evaluation of discussions, including the use of rubrics, and processing discussions with weekly synthesis weekly.
- Synthesize course discussions to summarize, reinforce, and give meaning to patterns being discussed in online courses.

As part of online discussions, questions serve as a way to engage students. Brookfield (2015) discussed teaching as a blend of conversations and questioning, noting the culture of inquiry promoted by questions. Although many questioning techniques used in the traditional classroom can be transferred to the online classroom, strategies such as wait time, eye contact, and tone are not available in text-based courses.

Online education presents a unique opportunity for enhancing the use of questions. Faculty can get a snapshot of students' thinking processes via questioning. Purposeful questions add an active component via approaches such as:

- Guiding student reflections on a particular topic. When questions are in the form of a student survey, for example, faculty can generate reports and then provide group feedback on the results or generate further questions for discussion.
- Summarizing responses to a clinical experience. Questions guide student reflections after clinical activities. For example, in a clinical course, students complete a summary and email it at the end of the clinical week responding to the following question: What is the best thing that happened? What was the most challenging thing?
- Guiding students with questions that help them reflect on what they are learning within specific modules. This approach adds an active learning component even to readings. Asking students to share three most important or interesting points for their practice from a reading supports learning of the community as well.

FEEDBACK TO STUDENTS ONLINE

Feedback in online education provides information about their achievements. Faculty-friendly ways exist to provide feedback in this unique learning medium. Whether feedback is part of a discussion, a sequenced progressive project, or brief assignment activities, it is a way to support learning and to promote student connection with the learning community. Appropriate feedback helps students gauge their learning progress and take further responsibility for their learning. Chapter 9 provides further information about feedback as a broad concept.

All online assignments are not created equal for feedback. Designing assignments with "fit" for good feedback and linking these assignments to course objectives are consistent with the Integrated Learning Triangle for Teaching With Technologies (Exhibit 1.3). Assignment design includes considering whether different types of feedback are needed at different points in the semester (perhaps related to maintaining course momentum and student learning). Other considerations include the following:

- Build student skills in seeking feedback, giving students permission to request additional feedback and guiding the best and most timely ways to access faculty.
- Designate selected assignments for the most focused feedback. For example, clarify with students that different types of assignments such as "learning activities" are for their own reflection and do not require extensive faculty feedback.
- Use templates for more efficiency in feedback. Automated grade books provide opportunities for timesaving templates that can be individualized with a brief phrase.
- Enhance opportunities for self-assessment, a type of self-feedback.
- Guide students in the use of rubrics to provide peer feedback on selected assignments.

Additional feedback issues in the course design phase include the pacing of the course assignments. Faculty will want to consider assignment depth and breadth, as well as time frame for completion of assignments and feedback. Major projects that build across the semester provide opportunities for multiple feedback opportunities before the product is finished. A faculty survey (Bonnel & Boehm, 2008) found that three broad categories of approaches guided faculty in efficient and effective ways to provide feedback:

- Having a system for feedback. Examples include being proactive and minimizing potential problems through early guidance and restating/clarifying expectations.
- Using best available tools. Examples include using rubrics, templates, and automated responses to assessing knowledge and increasing the efficiency of feedback response.
- Creating feedback-rich environments. Examples include use of assignments such as journal writing or self-assessment to stimulate students' self-examination and introspection to evaluate performance and stimulate critical thinking skills

An evidence-based review abstract is shared in Exhibit 10.5. This systematic review provides faculty direction for promoting online integrity.

EXHIBIT 10.5

EVIDENCE-BASED REVIEW ABSTRACT: SEEKING BEST EVIDENCE AND PROMOTING ONLINE INTEGRITY

Compiled by: Amanda L. Alonzo, PhD, RN

Challenge: Because an increasing number of nursing programs are developing online and web-enhanced formats, many faculty question the ability to ensure honesty and integrity in the online environment. Incorporating best practices in online honesty and integrity is essential to ensure the rigor of nursing education.

Sample best practices: Based on best literature evidence, best practices for promoting student honesty and integrity include using a log-in system particularly for online assessments, frequent faculty–student communication through email communication, discussion boards and chats to become familiar with individual students' writing style, incorporating a code of ethics in each course, using online software/websites to detect plagiarism in student work, and creating assignments to maximize student honesty and integrity.

Model case: A workshop was presented to expose faculty to best practices in promoting honesty and integrity in online learning and to provide an opportunity to use these strategies in assignments. Following a presentation on preventing plagiarism in written work, faculty worked on sample individual assignments to identify plagiarism and then worked on creating a sequenced progressive assignment designed to minimize opportunities for plagiarism.

Implications: Potential implications for implementing best practices in online honesty and integrity include faculty awareness and use of best practices, faculty experience in use of best-practice techniques, and increased student honesty and integrity.

Summary recommendations: Implementation of best practices in online honesty and integrity is essential for ensuring the quality of online nursing education. Through awareness of best literature evidence, nursing faculty will be better prepared to offer quality nursing education that promotes honesty and integrity in the online environment.

Strategies for proactively focusing on honesty in the online setting can help students focus on the positive ethical approaches to learning online.

CONTINUOUS QUALITY IMPROVEMENT AND ONLINE EDUCATION

As reflective educators, we take opportunities to look back at courses and assignments to determine what has and has not helped students learn in the online environment. We gain opportunities to revise or reshape the course components that are least successful. Consistent with the "Revise" component of the Integrated Learning Triangle for Teaching With Technologies (Exhibit 1.3), course continuous quality improvement (CQI) builds on this faculty reflection. For example, one author's evaluation practice typically includes seeking ongoing course module evaluations and student final semester evaluations with student activities throughout the semester (e.g., course project quality and student grades). Then, after reflecting on this information, relevant themes are noted and appropriate changes made to the course structure or process. Faculty course reflections can often lead to piloting of new teaching and learning strategies.

Ongoing module evaluations can provide rapid input from students as to what works in a course assignment or what does not. A useful tool for gaining quick student feedback on modules or assignments is asking students to complete fast-feedback forms (as an electronic survey within the modules), answering the following questions:

- What worked?
- What did not?
- What would you like to see changed?

Tools such as those developed by the Teaching, Learning, and Technology Group (2015) provide students with more formal opportunities to look back and rate the usefulness of an online course or assignment. Among other programs, the Quality Matters program is a faculty-centered, peer-review process designed to certify the quality of online courses and online components. The Quality Matters rubric consists of eight broad standards that identify desired outcomes and clarify acceptable evidence to show these course components are met including the following (Quality Matters, 2017):

1. Course overview and introduction
2. Learning objectives
3. Assessment and measurement
4. Resources and materials
5. Learner engagement
6. Course technology
7. Learner support
8. Accessibility

Further discussion is needed across nursing education that focuses on teaching best practices, evaluation, and CQI with online education; there is also a need to generate further research questions related to best practices. An example for discussion is massive open online courses (MOOCs). The philosophy of MOOCs is to provide, free via the Internet, interactive online courses to persons around the world from institutions such as Harvard University, Stanford University, and Massachusetts Institute of Technology. Although research on MOOCs is being generated, interest in them has expanded due to open access and anticipated further opportunities with MOOCs in higher education.

USING LEARNING MANAGEMENT SYSTEMS FOR ONLINE EDUCATION

Pedagogy and new technologies promote new ways of teaching and learning, with learning management systems as a major part of online learning. Further discussed in Chapters 9 and 11, they include features that can mimic the classroom. Useful features include the following online options:

- Distribute course materials.
- Post grades for students to access.
- Provide student surveys with tracking of online results.
- Interact with class participants via discussion boards or chat features.
- Create and administer tests or integrate with test software.

A focus on the learning and management functions in learning management systems provides enhanced teaching and learning opportunities. We want students to spend most of their time learning the content and not learning the technology. Facilitating optimal learning time includes focus on the following:

- Orienting students to the learning management system. Ideally, a technology support person will be available to students.
- Helping students be clear on what learning will be like online, addressing not only the learning management system, but also the process for learning in the course. This orientation can highlight the course roles of faculty and students, the types and purposes of varied assignments, and students' work as guided learners with self-directed emphasis. Orientations might be in the form of letters to students about the course or other online resources summarizing student guides. For example, instructors can begin a course with an audio presentation such as a voice-over PowerPoint or an Adobe-type synchronous session.

SUMMARY

Online education provides amazing opportunities to engage students in learning course concepts and to create enhanced learning using a world of resources. Faculty teaching strategies based on best practices include the concepts of design, facilitation, and feedback. A focus on beginnings, middles, and endings of courses provides further direction in course facilitation. Although face-to-face classroom learning and clinical experiences do not automatically come online, there are great opportunities for blending these approaches with online education.

ENDING REFLECTIONS FOR YOUR LEARNING NOTEBOOK

1. What is most important content that you learned in this chapter?
2. What are your plans for using the information provided in this chapter in your future teaching endeavors?
3. What are your further learning goals?

GUIDELINES FOR TEACHING AND LEARNING WITH TECHNOLOGIES

Quick Teaching Tips

1. Have a big picture of what should be accomplished in the course. Working backward in designing from the point of outcomes desired provides useful perspectives.
2. Consider how many ways real-world experiences can be incorporated into online readings and discussions.
3. Develop a learning community that provides students valued roles in self-assessment and peer review.

Questions for Further Reflection

1. Does being a good classroom teacher make you a good online teacher? What are similarities and differences?
2. What are the essential principles of good practice in online teaching? What examples of these principles come to mind for you to draw on?
3. What are the best ways to assess and engage diverse learning styles in online courses?
4. How is feedback different in online courses from that in face-to-face classes? In what ways do student and faculty roles specific to feedback change in the online setting? How do we know students are using and benefiting from feedback?
5. What are examples of strategies you use to promote self-assessment, peer review, and group work for feedback?

Learning Activity: Designing Opportunities for Online Feedback

The purpose of this activity is to design options for providing quality student feedback that is conducive to best teaching and learning practices.

Considering a course you are currently teaching (or would like to teach), how many of the following ways do you (or could you) integrate feedback into your online class?

Sample questions for each strategy (based on the type of course, level of students, and course objectives) include how to use the strategy, when to use it, how much weight to attach to it, and what is gained by this approach?

1. Self-evaluation/reflection
2. Groups assignments for feedback
3. Peer-critique strategies
4. Feedback from others (mentors/course guests)
5. Automated feedback with rubrics
6. Feedback from faculty

Online Resources for Further Learning

- ■ *Quality Matters.* This is a resource for professional development, building community, rubrics, and standards. www.qualitymatters.org
- ■ *MOOCs.* This resource compares and contrasts the best MOOC platforms. www.reviews.com/mooc-platforms

REFERENCES

Benner, P., Tanner, C., & Chesla, C. (Eds.). (2009). *Expertise in nursing practice: caring, clinical judgment, and ethics* (2nd ed.). New York, NY: Springer Publishing.

Boettcher, J. V. (2011). Designing for learning: Ten best practices for teaching online: Quick guide for new online faculty. Retrieved from http://www.designingforlearning.info/services/writing/ecoach/tenbest.html

Bonnel, W., & Boehm, H. (2011). Improving feedback to students online: Teaching tips from experienced faculty. *Journal of Continuing Education in Nursing, 42*(11), 503–509. doi:10.3928/00220124-20110715-02

Bonnel, W., & Meek, (2007). Qualitative assignments to enhance online learning communities. *Instructional Technology and Distance Learning, 4*(2), 49–54. Retrieved from http://www.itdl.org/journal/feb_07/article04.htm

Brookfield, S. (2015). *The skillful teacher: On technique, trust, and responsiveness in the classroom* (3rd ed). San Francisco, CA: Jossey Bass.

Carnegie Mellon University. (2015). Principles of teaching. Retrieved from https://www.cmu.edu/teaching/principles/teaching.html

Chickering, A. W., & Ehrmann, S. C. (1996). Implementing the seven principles: Technology as lever. *AAHE Bulletin, 49*, 3–6. Retrieved from http://www.iupui.edu/~cletcrse/ncaa/seven.htm

Fink, L. D. (2013). *Creating significant learning experiences: An integrated approach to designing college courses* (2nd ed.). San Francisco, CA: Jossey-Bass.

Hanover Research Council. (2009). Best practices in online teaching strategies. Retrieved from http://www.uwec.edu/AcadAff/resources/edtech/upload/Best-Practices-in-Online-Teaching-Strategies-Membership.pdf

McKeachie, W., & Svinicki, M. (2014). Problem-based learning: Teaching with cases, simulations, and games. In W. McKeachie & M. Svinicki (Eds.), *McKeachie's teaching tips: Strategies, research, and theory for college and university teachers* (14th ed.). Boston, MA: Houghton Mifflin.

National Academy of Sciences. (2015). *Reaching students: What research says about effective instruction in undergraduate science and engineering*. Retrieved from https://www.nap.edu/catalog/18687/reaching-students-what-research-says-about-effective-instruction-in-undergraduate

O'Neil, C. (2014). Reconceptualizing the online course. In C. O'Neil, C. Fisher, & M. Rietschel (Eds.), *Developing online learning environments in nursing education* (3rd ed., pp. 61–72). New York, NY: Springer Publishing.

Palloff, R. M., & Pratt, K. (2001). *Lessons from the cyberspace classroom: The realities of online teaching*. San Francisco, CA: Jossey-Bass.

Quality Matters. (2017). The quality matters rubric. Retrieved from https://www.qualitymatters.org/qa-resources/rubric-standards

The Teaching, Learning, and Technology Group (2015). Vision worth working toward anthology. Retrieved from http://www.tltgroup.org/anthology

Weimer, M. (2013). *Learner-centered teaching: Five key changes to practice* (2nd ed.). San Francisco, CA: Jossey-Bass.

CHAPTER 11

Hybrid Learning: The Changing Classroom and Technology to Promote Quality Care

CHAPTER GOAL

Gain strategies for using technology in the changing classroom to promote student learning for safety and quality in patient care.

BEGINNING REFLECTION

1. What have been your most positive recent experiences with the changing classroom and technologies? What have been the most challenging experiences?
2. What goals do you have for further use of technologies in promoting quality care in the changing classroom?

Overheard: *I heard that flipped classrooms are the preferred teaching strategy of the future, but I am not sure how they work.*

Changes in student populations, more rapid proliferation of information, and more technology resources lead to the use of the classroom in new ways. In the past, faculty may have had huge notebooks of information they verbally imparted to students. Now students access online presentations and create additional learning tips via combinations of lecture and Internet reviews. For some faculty, the changing classroom means using clickers or automated response systems (ARS); for others it means bringing real-time video of simulations to students in the classroom. Technology is changing our use of the classroom, including different approaches to space, time, and hands versus fingertip learning (Verkuyl, Romaniuk, Atack, & Mastrilli, 2017).

In traditional classrooms, students were passive learners or class participants. Research on how people learn supports the finding that people learn best by being actively engaged, and different tools or technologies work best for achieving this (Commission on Behavioral and Social Sciences and Education, 1999). As students change from being the passive classroom learner, they encounter many technologies that bring opportunities for extending active learning roles and outcomes. Technology can also increase ties to clinical experiences by bringing clinical cases and virtual experiences into the classroom using mobile devices (Skiba, 2017). The question then becomes how to best use technologies to achieve an effective balance or blend of classroom support and learning challenges.

Changing the classroom may present initial challenges related to the more traditional teaching models in which students expected their teachers to take the stage and provide a lecture. Weimer (2013) describes the changing function of course content, describing content as an opportunity for learning engagement and suggesting that it be used in class rather than merely covered. For example, the incorporation of active teaching strategies requires students to search, decide, and build for connections to case studies, stories, and patient care plans. This shift promotes students' self-awareness as learners, their understanding of how they learn, and their ability to learn more as they gain new skill sets. Benner, Tanner, and Chesla (2009) note, for example, that cases and questions help move classroom theory to patient care in the clinical setting. This chapter describes strategies for combining the best of the traditional teaching and learning strategies with new rapidly changing technologies.

Although faculty no longer need a real-world classroom to teach a course or even give a lecture, there are advantages to a physical classroom. Students bring diverse interests and reasons for being there. The classroom brings historical perspectives (the familiarity of the learning setting that most students grew up with). It also offers pedagogical opportunities that can be enhanced with technology. The classroom setting may be particularly important for beginning learners. In the classroom, faculty have the opportunity to personalize learning, convey enthusiasm, model critical thinking, and enliven text-based information (Bradshaw & Lowenstein, 2016). Additional classroom benefits include the following:

- There can be an intensity or intimacy of learning. Faculty and students have the advantage of face-to-face conversations and can gain the immediate feel of a community.
- Faculty have more opportunities for modeling professional behaviors. We can read the body language of students. Clarifications in communications or follow-up questions can immediately occur.

Faculty use the classroom in different ways at different times. Students come to classrooms with different knowledge and mental sets at different points in time. As we think about our pedagogies for helping students move from backgrounds of limited knowledge to skill sets for managing complex patient care, we may need to put additional focus on Benner's (2001) novice to expert transitions. Different teaching technologies may be needed at different points for different student skill sets to best support students.

Technology allows us to easily bring active learning into the classroom by using strategies such as student self-assessments, applied case studies, quiz questions embedded in PowerPoint presentations, and projects with clinical applications. Examples of clinical applications are evidence-based posters or patient care materials that use the content in authentic ways. The remaining content in this chapter provides an overview of interactive learning opportunities with technology in the classroom, the classroom as an opportunity for extending distance learning, and the role of learning management systems.

TOOLS FOR INTERACTIVE LEARNING

Research has long established that students learn more, understand what they learn more deeply, and retain information longer when they are engaged in their own learning tasks (Commission on Behavioral and Social Sciences and Education, 1999). Higher-order thinking happens when motivated students connect information, content, and skills from courses to real-world situations (Fink, 2013). A key component of a successful course is to have a teacher who can think innovatively and facilitate active student engagement in the subject matter and the learning process.

Principles that have been widely used as a framework for evaluating teaching quality draw from the "Seven Principles for Good Practice in Undergraduate Education" by Chickering and Gamson (1987). Another principle for consideration in quality teaching practices is to effectively integrate technologies (Cable and Cheung, 2017). We, as educators, need to continually explore new learning tools and strategies to support teaching, deciding on course areas to improve by using one or two new technology applications, such as automated response systems, PowerPoint, and flipped classroom strategies.

Automated Response Systems or Clickers in the Classroom

Automated response systems, sometimes referred to as clickers, classroom response, or ARS, have practical and critical relevance to 21st century learning systems. Clicker-like teaching strategies are used in case studies, opinion polls, and quizzes, encouraging active student participation in content review. Chien, Chang, and Chang (2017) found that clickers seem to positively impact student cognition, motivation, and behavior during learning. Interestingly, clicker activities engage student self-regulatory processes that monitor the gap between actual and desired performance, encouraging students to proactively seek and interpret information, and peer discussions impact the performance-feedback-adjustment loop. Clicker-integrated instruction is positively associated with meeting academic learning outcomes.

EXHIBIT 11.1

EVIDENCE-BASED REVIEW ABSTRACT: LISTENING FOR A "CLICK" IN CLASSROOMS

Compiled by Shelley D. Barenklau, CRNA, DNP

Automated response systems using clicker remotes promote active learning and support classroom communication within a variety of academic settings. *Clickers* have re-entered classrooms to increase student participation, expand discussion, and challenge students to assess their level of understanding using an immediate feedback system. A literature review was conducted to examine best-practice guidelines for implementing and using ARS in graduate classrooms, specifically examining ARS use in nurse anesthesia education. A variety of goals and uses for ARS emerged from review of the literature: increasing classroom interactivity, inclusive classroom participation, increased attention spans, formative assessment, peer learning, and assessment of student accountability. Overall, references suggest that clickers positively contribute to student comprehension, improved test scores, and satisfaction. Scientific conclusions for best-practice guidelines for ARS are still emerging, and further research is indicated because many existing references are experiential in nature. Clickers may prove key to improving test scores or may merely be a fun and innovative method to capture student attention and generate classroom interaction. The answer remains a "click" away.

ARS, automated response systems.

There are as many ways to use clickers as there are to frame different types of survey and quiz questions, varying from agree/disagree responses to multiple choice. Relevant to broad content and process topics, clickers give students the opportunity to review course material and to practice test-taking in preparation for standardized examinations. They also provide faculty with snapshot assessments of students' knowledge. An evidence-based review abstract on automated response systems is provided in Exhibit 11.1. Finding the right balance of clicker use may be an issue with further research needed on this topic.

Active Learning and PowerPoint: Making the Lecture Interactive

Active learning and PowerPoint are a good mix when combined for interactive classroom presentation. An interactive PowerPoint builds in reminders for interaction with students. There has been debate about PowerPoint use in the classroom, with some educators suggesting that the tool creates passive learners. In the past, PowerPoint presentations gained a reputation for being long bulleted lists of topical information that, although informative, were often difficult for students to retain. When coupled with active learning activities that engage the audience, however, bulleted information lists are better retained. Asking students, for example, to apply selected bullets to a brief case application provides an enhanced learning opportunity. The interactive lecture not only organizes content, highlighting the "must know" information, but also engages students in learning the information (Bradshaw & Lowenstein, 2016). PowerPoint uses include the following:

- Meets the needs of diverse learners, providing opportunities to engage their hearing and visual senses, thus engaging students with both auditory and visual learning preferences.
- Addresses the needs of visual learners with the visual benefits of PowerPoint in terms of showing diagrams and concept relationships. There are good opportunities for visual cues and opportunity to focus on the visual benefits, such as providing a wound picture for students to assess and then asking students to document their findings.
- Provides a structure for organizing learning concepts, helping faculty remain organized in classroom presentations. It provides learners with neat, legible notes, supporting both prior reading and in-class note taking.
- Serves as a strategy for engaging the audience. Changing the pace of the presentation with an active learning approach can be a useful strategy for keeping students engaged.

When using interactive lectures, with PowerPoint or automated response systems, active learning opportunities can be provided. A good beginning question for faculty to consider is, "How am I using PowerPoint and is it to everyone's advantage?" Examples of various PowerPoint strategies for engaging learners are included in Exhibit 11.2 All of these approaches are amenable for use with automated response systems or raising of hands in response to questions.

WEB-BASED MODULES AS A CLASSROOM ADJUNCT

The Internet can be used for education and teaching on almost any topic. Commonly referred to as a blended classroom, the result is a combination of the physical classroom with an online learning space to improve education for students (see Exhibit 11.3 to learn from a practicing educator). As Kathleen Ward, Faculty Champion, explains in Exhibit 11.3, incorporating a blended classroom requires time and commitment. Ward encourages faculty to start small, incorporating one or two aspects of the blended classroom per semester while periodically assessing student learning outcomes such as satisfaction, motivation, and knowledge acquisition.

Products such as web-based review modules can also provide benefits in blended classrooms. Using the Internet to provide supplementary (or required) healthcare information can be a time-efficient approach for educators. The online classroom is useful particularly as we seek to have students be prepared for classroom sessions and want to challenge them to use concepts postclass.

EXHIBIT 11.2

SAMPLE ACTIVE LEARNING OPPORTUNITIES FOR INTERACTIVE POWERPOINT PRESENTATIONS

Cases: Cases are a good way to illustrate points being made on an earlier slide. They promote retention because it is often easier to remember cases than a list of bulleted facts. Combining the two is a good strategy.

Stories: Stories of clinical practice help tie concepts/theory to practice. There is limited teaching value, for example, if content taught is not used/modeled in clinical settings. How best to use technology to help student's gain and transfer information from classroom to clinical setting will be an ongoing challenge that technologies such as video, simulation, and telehealth may help to answer.

Reflective prompts and discussion questions: Active learning activities can include discussion opportunities during PowerPoint presentations. After broad key points on a topic are covered, pertinent questions/prompts to promote reflection and use of the content can lead to further discussion. Key themes from the discussion can be noted.

Multiple choice: Multiple-choice practice test questions can be used as a review for an upcoming exam. Students have an opportunity to learn from one another as they discuss the correct answer and provide explanations for incorrect responses.

Pair/share activities: General guides for pair/share activities include providing a question, asking student pairs to discuss the question for two minutes, and then calling on selected groups to summarize their discussion.

Organizing cues: Organized PowerPoint handouts are helpful in student learning, especially when used with the required reading. In a pathophysiology course, for example, it would be appropriate to suggest reviewing the PowerPoint handouts prior to class, making additional notes in the margins from information gathered from readings.

Surveys/debriefing: Stopping the class for an opinion poll on a specific question with potential for multiple perspectives promotes critical thinking and reflection.

EXHIBIT 11.3

TIPS FROM FACULTY CHAMPIONS: BLENDED CLASSROOMS TIPS FROM A CHAMPIONS' Q&A

Kathleen Ward, MSN, RN

1. *What is your current position like, relevant to implementing blended classrooms? What formal or informal education or training have you had in blended classrooms?* My current faculty position lends itself to the implementation of blended classroom activities. I use some form of blended learning in all of my courses. All of my education in blended classroom activities has been acquired through reading research articles, attending various education conferences, and reading web-based offerings. I challenge myself to learn about a new technique or strategy and then transform it to a specific course objective.

2. *What are the key points related to teaching and learning needs for blended classrooms that faculty would need to better understand?* Technological knowledge is key when considering the use of the blended classroom. Most faculty did not grow up in a

(continued)

technologically rich environment. In addition, the advances in software that avail themselves to a blended classroom environment have also grown exponentially, leaving many faculty unsure of which ones to try. Free and low-cost software or software purchased by the institution are excellent places to start. Incorporating this concept into the classroom requires time and commitment. It is best to start small, incorporating one or two aspects of the blended classroom, then building in subsequent semesters. This method also allows the faculty member time to assess this teaching modality on a more random number of students.

3. **How do you manage to keep a student-focused learning approach using blended classrooms? What ways do you see your faculty or students benefiting from better understanding blended classrooms?** Keeping students focused and engaged in a blended classroom is easier than in the traditional classroom. When students can use the technology on their cell phones or computers they come alive; they interact, communicate, and learn. Students help fellow classmates learn when using texting on their cell phones to discuss the rationales for the answers to the questions. But remember to develop guidelines for blended classroom activities. Research has shown that students learn and retain more when engaged in the learning; for this reason, I believe it is important for faculty to incorporate this concept. It is rewarding to the faculty member when students truly understand the content. Students also feel a sense of accomplishment when completing the task.

4. *What are select facilitators for incorporating blended classrooms into your nursing education courses/programs?* Key processes for incorporating the blended classroom concept into my courses are as follows: First and foremost, get buy-in and support from the upper administration. Second is the availability of technology in the classroom; our technologically enriched classrooms enable themselves uniquely for this concept. The biggest challenge is the time factor. I am constantly working on incorporating or building on methods to use within all of my courses. Researching and revising a concept to fit uniquely to my content takes time. In addition, I have to continually reevaluate what I already have in place.

5. *In what ways do you use blended classrooms to help students learn about safety and/or quality management for clinical settings?* In my practicum courses I use the individual rotation strategy, which is an excellent approach to helping student appreciate safety and quality management and use it in the clinical setting. Students partake in the individualized rotation experience in a simulated setting and afterward complete an online learning activity. The online learning activity is my current blended classroom work in progress.

6. *What is your favorite assignment for a student-focused learning approach in your teaching? How do you manage to stay creative with your approaches?* My favorite assignment for student-focused learning requires students to use a free app wherein they can create their own actors and scene and write their script to construct a video. They can add emotions, sound effects, and music. The assignment requires the student to develop growth and development teaching on the basis of their assigned patient age range and task. After selecting their actors and scenes, they type in the teaching that they would provide to parents about what growth and developmental tasks their child should be achieving during this period. When all the teaching projects are completed, students are required to review everyone's video and complete the online assignment.

7. *What tips or advice would you like to share with new faculty teaching in a blended classroom?* Research the topic, attend educational offerings on the topic, and then start. Start small, ***but start!*** One class, one assignment, or activity at a time. This is a rewarding experience not only for the students, but also for the faculty member. You will feel a sense of accomplishment while using technology in one of blended classroom modalities. At the end, it can make your job easier while students learn and retain more of the content.

One type of blended classroom found in the literature is the flipped classroom. As Brame (2013) explains, an inverted or flipped classroom is a teaching pedagogy in which students are expected to gain first exposure to theory content before coming to class by completing assignments, including readings, lecture videos, and/or PowerPoint presentations with voice-over. This "preparatory" knowledge and content gain are intended to later facilitate higher forms of cognitive processing (such as analyzing, problem-solving, and debating) in class with the support of peers and the instructor.

Three key elements for implementing the flipped classroom include an incentive for student class preparation; mechanisms to assess student understanding before, during, and/or after class; and in-class activities that focus on higher-level cognitive activities, such as case studies, that actively and interactively clarify and apply knowledge during class. Although more research examining the outcomes of the flipped classroom is needed, studies currently support flipped classrooms for student-centered learning and collaboration with technology applications for team, problem-based, and case-based healthcare practice (Betihavas, Bridgman, Kornhaber, & Cross, 2016).

Comprehensively, a virtual tour provides a package of educational materials based on web resources that students can use to learn the materials now and to keep as a resource for future review. Used as tools to build on students' current knowledge levels, virtual tours can be quickly skimmed brief modules or more detailed modules for enhanced learning. For example, after a class on the care of patients with dementia, students may not recall all the unique facts of family caregiving with dementia patients, but they can likely recall a good web-based resource for future use. Access to the website for support group resources and patient education information provides a useful clinical tool. As students continue to access the Alzheimer's Association website, they will also find the most current information, including updates on treatments and research.

Virtual tours can be used as a type of homework or for preclass or postclass discussion preparation. Also, to extend independent learning, students can be asked to become familiar with the Internet resources that have topical information on specialty topics of interest (e.g., parish nursing resources, evidence-based summaries from organizations such as those focused on palliative care).

TECHNOLOGY FOR MANAGING CLASSROOMS: LEARNING MANAGEMENT SYSTEMS

Although this book is about pedagogies for teaching with technologies, it is worthwhile to also consider the management functions provided by technology in the classroom. Learning management systems are tools, such as Blackboard, that make it easier to organize our classes. They provide a variety of ways to manage classroom activities, including communication, distribution of course materials, and grading. Instead of copying volumes of information for students and carrying it to classrooms, we can now develop and organize our class documents in learning management systems. Students can print what they want and use electronic versions as they need, easily accessing class notes, class study guides, and other resources. Examples of options include the following:

- Using learning management systems for organizing grades
- Providing additional resources and websites for review
- Providing practice tests and online reviews
- Offering opportunities for student surveys
- Analyzing items on tests
- Providing course calendars with assignment due dates and study and project guides

Basic communication features of learning management systems such as announcement features, email, and discussion boards promote enhanced communication with and between students. These collection resources for student assignments enhance opportunities for providing feedback and making grades easily accessible to students. As we seek efficient, effective education, learning management systems provide tools to accomplish classroom management tasks.

Classroom management is enhanced with these tools, but they also help faculty facilitate learning with good pedagogical principles. Promoting and supporting learning uses best practices with learning management systems, as introduced in earlier chapters. Assignments and project activities can be incorporated in new ways with tools such as discussion boards, blogs, and Wikis for group sharing. Many benefits can be obtained with these tools if they are used as more than receptacles for delivering and receiving class materials. Sample strategies enhanced within the learning management system include the following:

- Organizing students into groups for project work or discussions, learning management systems provide ways to extend assignment and classroom discussions, whether synchronous or asynchronous. To summarize readings, students might have discussion boards where they are assigned to share the three most interesting things they learned from readings.
- Another strategy is to provide preclass assignments from which faculty can select examples to share and build on during class. For example, question can be posted online so that students can respond to them prior to class. Answers and examples allow opportunities for faculty to share personal student examples that quickly involve their diverse students. A similar approach can have students share case examples or experiences, such as previous work with particular patient populations.
- In addition, technology can be used to guide students' informal writing to promote learning in larger classes, such as using slide prompts to encourage summary notes (or further questions to explore) as the class progresses

ALTERNATE CLASSROOM EXPERIENCE FOR STUDENTS AT A DISTANCE

Distance education has a long history and has even changed the ways that we think about classrooms. There are now tools available, such as classroom capture, online lecture, and interactive online voice-over PowerPoint classes, for our work with students. These unique opportunities take representations of the classroom to the students. Distance education literature (Viberg & Grönlund, 2015) has provided guidance in making classroom-type opportunities available to students at sites distant from the traditional classroom. In reviewing the following technologies that provide opportunities for distance education, it is useful to consider which of the traditional classroom strategies are most beneficial to retain in distance learning. For example, although lecture can be used in these formats as a teaching strategy, traditional lecture formats can create passive learners.

What are some of the approaches that attempt to provide a classroom setting at a distance when our students do not come to the traditional classroom? The classroom moves to multipoint conferencing software, such as Elluminate-type programs or Camtasia (merging tools for screen capture, audio–video recording to provide the effect of classroom capture).

- *Web-conferencing software*: Products such as Elluminate, Blackboard Collaborate Ultra, and Zoom provide faculty with real-time presentation opportunities with live group web discussions, sharing white boards, presentation software, and other tools. Students and faculty have the opportunity to communicate in real time verbally or in writing.
- *Classroom capture software*: If students do not come to class (for whatever reason) classroom capture software exists that can provide much of the classroom experience as the student watches a video of the class.
- *Audio casts*: Tools to create podcasts and voice-over PowerPoint provide unidirectional audio broadcasts that promote opportunity for a more traditional lecture. Creative thinking with PowerPoint presentations (as noted above) provides faculty opportunities to promote an engaging climate with these presentations.
- *Interactive television (ITV)*: Faculty and students seek strategies to connect with others at a distance, so teaching and learning are extended to multiple classrooms via ITV (or the receiving and sending of audio and video via an Internet protocol address). ITV allows large real-time classrooms at distant sites to be engaged for interaction with faculty. In addition, desktop or web camera applications exist for a variety of conferencing systems for individual desktop conferencing and small conference rooms.

With any of the visual mediums, good pedagogy includes focus on positive use of both verbal and nonverbal cues in classroom presentations. Verbal cues include, for example, accepting and reacting to students' emotions, providing positive reinforcement, giving appropriate classroom feedback to students, and using questioning as a learning tool. Positive nonverbal cues such as eye contact, facial expressions, posture, and energy level help convey content as do appropriate use of gestures, mannerisms, and movement in the classroom.

Students using any of these resources might gain information from some type of presentation as a tool for learning advanced practice nursing care. A statewide collaborative in Kansas, for example (V. Yu, personal communication, December 6, 2017), brings opportunity to share expertise from practitioners across the state via a statewide repository of lectures and interactive learning materials. Students across the state learn in their homes as clinical experts share voice-over PowerPoint presentations on varied topics, as well as provide interactive content quizzes and assignments. As a result, healthcare is transformed as traditional theory content is professionally shared using integrated, context-relevant, useful technologies.

Additional technologies can be used in connection with these tools to create learning communities that provide a more social feel of the classroom. For example, professional networking sites similar to social sites such as Facebook and LinkedIn present potential for building professional peer involvement. Young (2016) describes the benefits of sharing professionally in a specialty area within these communities and describes low-cost options.

SUMMARY

The teaching methods that we choose for our courses depend on our goals for learning. The classroom provides unique opportunities for learning with technology. Learning in a classroom setting is a revered and often practical way to promote student knowledge gain. For many years faculty lectures, or telling students about content, has been the typical classroom approach. Now, technology provides the changing classroom with opportunities for enhanced learning through interactive content applications. Technology in the changing classroom provides opportunities to combine the best of traditional and new teaching approaches.

ENDING REFLECTIONS FOR YOUR LEARNING NOTEBOOK

1. What is the most important content that you learned in this chapter?
2. What are your plans for using the information provided in this chapter in your future teaching endeavors?
3. What are your further learning goals?

GUIDELINES FOR TEACHING AND LEARNING WITH TECHNOLOGIES

Quick Teaching Tips

1. Keep the classroom interactive with varied technologies such as clickers and pair/share activities.
2. If using PowerPoint, include reminder slides for interactive activities to break up a lecture.
3. Ask students to complete electronic fast-feedback forms following class to indicate what they learned that was most useful and what they still have questions about.

Questions for Further Reflection

1. What makes the classroom unique for beginning students compared with advanced students? Are there best practices for technology in the classroom depending on student level?
2. How can learning management systems best be used for the pedagogical opportunities as well as management perspectives?

Learning Activity: Can PowerPoint Be Used for Active Learning?

The purpose of this activity is to decide if using PowerPoint is an appropriate teaching methodology in a given learning context or situation. In making this decision, reflect on which of the following slides (or combinations) might help accomplish student learning objectives for a class you plan to teach:

1. Specific slides that remind students what they have done to prepare for class (e.g., preassignments such as readings, pretests or student reflections about their own experiences related to the topic)
2. Specific slides that remind you to create "set" for the class (e.g., "This is what we are going to accomplish today" or "Some of the things we will be doing include....")
3. Specific slides that remind you to include active learning opportunities (e.g., reminders for you to stop and engage students using techniques such as true/false questions, case studies, pair/share activities, and other learning activities that help students engage with the content being taught, or a simple reminder slide with the word "questions?")
4. Preclass or postclass sharing of experiences or observations
5. Periodic summary slides (e.g., "So far this is what we've learned...")
6. Specific slide reminding you to bring closure to the lesson (e.g., the high points covered)
7. A student "challenge" slide to consider how they might start using the content right away. Additional assignments...or a slide that simple asks "What next?"

Online Resources for Further Learning

- Distance Education for Teacher Training. This resource provides online tools for technology modes, education models, and instructional methods. idd.edc.org/sites/idd.edc.org/files/Distance%20Education%20for%20Teacher%20Training%20by%20Mary%20Burns%20EDC.pdf
- International Society for Technology in Education (ISTE) standards. This online community is dedicated to learning the skills and knowledge necessary to rethink education within a constantly changing technological landscape. www.iste.org/standards

REFERENCES

Benner, P. (2001). *From novice to expert, commemorative edition*. Upper Saddle River, NJ: Prentice Hall Health.

Benner, P., Tanner, C., & Chesla, C. (Eds.). (2009). *Expertise in nursing practice: Caring, clinical judgment, and ethics* (2nd ed.). New York, NY: Springer Publishing.

Betihavas, V., Bridgman, H., Kornhaber, R., & Cross, M. (2016). The evidence for "flipping out": A systematic review of the flipped classroom in nursing education. *Nurse Education Today, 38*, 15–21. doi:10.1016/j.nedt.2015.12.010

Bradshaw, M., & Lowenstein, A. (2016). *Innovative teaching strategies in nursing & related health professions* (7th ed.). Sudbury, MA: Jones & Bartlett.

Brame, C. (2013). Flipping the classroom. Vanderbilt University Center for Teaching. Retrieved from https://cft.vanderbilt.edu/guides-sub-pages/flipping-the-classroom

Cable, J., & Cheung, C. (2017). Eight principles of effective online teaching: A decade-long lessons learned in project management education. *PM Journal, 6*(7), 1–16. Retrieved from https://pmworldjournal.net/article/eight-principles-effective-online-teaching/

Chickering, A., & Gamson, Z. (1987). Seven principles for good practice in undergraduate education. *AAHE Bulletin, 39*, 3–7. Retrieved from https://files.eric.ed.gov/fulltext/ED282491.pdf

Chien, Y.-T., Chang, Y.-H., & Chang, C.-Y. (2017). Do we click in the right way? A meta-analytic review of clicker-integrated instruction. *Educational Research Review, 17*, 1–18. doi:10.1016/j.edurev.2015.10.003

Commission on Behavioral and Social Sciences and Education. (1999). *How people learn: Bridging research and practice*. Washington, DC: National Academies Press. Retrieved from http://www.nap.edu/catalog.php?record_id=9457

Fink, L. D. (2013). *Creating significant learning experiences: An integrated approach to designing college courses* (2nd ed.). San Francisco, CA: Jossey-Bass

Verkuyl, M., Romaniuk, D., Atack, L., & Mastrilli, P. (2017). Virtual gaming simulation for nursing education: An experiment. *Clinical Simulation in Nursing, 13*, 238–244. doi:10.1016/j.ecns.2017.02.004

Viberg, O., & Grönlund, A. (2015). Understanding students' learning practices: Challenges for design and integration of mobile technology into distance education. *Learning, Media, and Technology, 42*(3), 357–377. doi:10.1080/17439884.2016.1088869

Weimer, M. (2013). *Learner-centered teaching: Five key changes to practice* (2nd ed.). San Francisco, CA: Jossey-Bass.

Young, J. R. (2016). The story of a digital teddy bear shows how college learning is changing. Retrieved from https://www.chronicle.com/article/The-Story-of-a-Digital-Teddy/234881

CHAPTER 12

Simulation: Creating Safe Environments for Learning Patient Care

CHAPTER GOAL

Gain a variety of ideas on how to incorporate simulation into students' clinical learning experiences.

BEGINNING REFLECTION

1. How can simulation provide a safe environment in which students learn to meet clinical competencies?
2. What experiences have you had with high-fidelity patient simulation?
3. What is your familiarity with gaming and the best strategies for its implementation in the curriculum?

Overheard: *They told me I have to teach with simulation. I am not so sure about this.*

How does technology relate to clinical learning? Clinical practice is a fundamental element of nursing, so teaching students to apply didactic content and skills to competent clinical practice is an essential element of their education. In the past, clinical skills were learned and practiced on live people. Although that approach provided necessary real-life experience, it also left concerns about the quality of care received by some patients, the ethical implications of practicing on people, and the problem that not all students had the same opportunity to experience the same clinical situations.

Advances in technology have led to methods that mitigate these concerns about clinical education. Students can now have virtual experiences that create the opportunity to learn a wide variety of specific clinical skills, as well as exercise the critical thinking skills necessary in live situations, without the potential risk of harming real patients. In these created situations or scenarios, students play the role of a healthcare provider to simulated patients (a manne-quin or computer character, for example) in fictitious settings (e.g., a hospital room or a community clinic). Technology thus creates a means to provide clinical learning for all students, which is safe, effective, and standardized.

Another advantage of simulations is that all students can experience the same clinical situations. Because the simulated experiences are fictitious, they can be created repeatedly at any time, so that faculty and students are not dependent on what happens (or does not happen) at an actual clinical site. A faculty member who wants all students to run a code, help with labor, or resuscitate an infant can develop a scenario and use high-fidelity patient simulation (HFPS) to ensure that all students get that specific experience. Simulation offers not only an effective method for learning these lessons, but also an efficient method for evaluating students' formative and summative learning.

In addition to creating a safer learning environment and standardizing clini-cal learning experiences for all students, simulation also provides an opportunity for educational experiences based on the best practices and sound educational theories. Being placed in a simulated scenario reinforces the immediate appli-cation of content suggested in adult education theory, the active participation of learners necessary to create meaning in constructivist theory, and the multiple intricacies of clinical situations in which students will practice as suggested in complexity theory. Although the exact technological means to do so will con-tinue to change, an overview of simulation-based education and basic principles of simulation use are presented, followed by two current examples (HFPS and virtual world electronic gaming) of simulation use in healthcare education.

OVERVIEW OF SIMULATION-BASED EDUCATION

Although there are many simulation options, in this book we focus on HFPS and electronic gaming in the virtual world of Second Life. Simulators are devices that recreate characteristics of the real world, and simulation fidel-ity is the degree to which they do so successfully (Beaubien & Baker, 2004). Low-fidelity simulators are not as lifelike as high-fidelity simulators. Today's HFPSs, although still bearing a resemblance to the mannequins of days gone by, are much more refined in that they blink; breathe; urinate; have ECGs, blood pressures and heart rhythms; and respond in physiologically appropri-ate ways to dose-specific medications. These mannequins are available in the shapes and sizes of infant, child, adult, and laboring woman. There are a num-ber of manufactures, and each varies in exactly what their respective HFPS offers. For example, students cannot suction a tracheostomy or provide gas-trostomy tube feeding and care on some HFPSs but can on others. Similarly, some HFPS products offer central-line catheter site care, dressing changes, infusions, and line flushing, but others do not. Faculty should know what they need and ask appropriate questions.

HFPS scenarios are very lifelike. They are written to address specific topical content and are directed by the specific learning outcomes and objectives for the HFPS learning experience. The scenario is set up in a physical room that might mimic a hospital room, an operating room, an outpatient clinic, or a patient's home. The HFPS generally fills the patient role, and students generally play the nurse in the scenario, although all sorts of variations have been used. As the scenario progresses, students are physically present as they interact with the HFPS, make decisions, and provide care.

At the same time HFPS has become more technologically advanced, students are growing up using computer-based games and virtual worlds that offer potential benefits to healthcare education as well. *Electronic games* refer to interactive games provided via digital technology and, although many of the early games were for pure entertainment, their potential has now turned to the training of healthcare professionals who can now be immersed in real-life situations in which they must think and act accordingly. Although still technically gaming, this practice is now considered as *virtual serious games* (Verkuyl, Romaniuk, Atack, & Mastrilli, 2017) or virtual worlds.

Although gaming for pleasure may not be foreign to us, the idea of inserting ourselves—not as a generic game character but as a character using one's own thoughts, decisions, and actions—into that virtual world may feel less natural. Whatever the virtual setting—hospital, community clinic, or patient's home or neighborhood—people in that setting use avatars to play themselves. Electronic gaming is really a natural extension of the human simulator. With HFPS, students are physically inserted into a scenario in which they interact with patients and other healthcare providers. In gaming the student represents him/herself as an avatar and is inserted into a virtual world where he/she interacts virtually with the patient and other healthcare providers.

BASIC PRINCIPLES OF USING SIMULATION

There are good resources for guiding your work using simulation in your teaching and learning activities. The Standards of Best Practice: Simulation were developed by the International Nursing Association for Clinical Simulation and Learning (INACSL; 2016) to provide and share evidence-based guidelines for use in simulation. The standards include the following content areas: simulation design, outcomes and objectives, facilitation, debriefing, participant evaluation, professional integrity, simulation-enhanced interprofessional education (IPE), and simulation glossary. Each standard includes background information for context, as well as required criteria and elements for meeting each standard.

Learning Outcomes and Objectives

As with any learning activity, the instructor must assess learners' needs to determine the appropriate activity based on the learners themselves, the learning experience objectives, and available resources. For example, you must be sure you know the knowledge level and experiences students bring to the simulation so that you write scenario objectives at the right level. You must also be clear on the intended scenario outcomes, so that the scenario itself is designed to enable students to achieve those outcomes.

Using the correct resources is critical. If the goal is to teach cardiopulmonary resuscitation techniques with first-semester clinical students, for example, then you would likely forgo using the HFPS in favor of the more basic Resusci Anne. On the other hand, if the goal is to teach arrhythmias and cardiac monitoring with third-semester clinical students, then you might create a scenario in which a patient's heart and breathing stop, with this event serving as a catalyst for the rest of the scenario. In this case, you may opt for the HFPS so that the ECG can be easily monitored and the rhythms changed as needed. You should match the scenario design to the learning goals, participants, scenario objectives, and most appropriate resources. You should keep in mind that a number of sources (including two resources by the National League for Nursing [NLN]: Simulation Innovation Resource Center [SIRC] and Advancing Care Excellence for Seniors [ACES]) have already developed cases that can be used as is or can be modified to meet your specific outcomes and objectives.

Rubrics

Once goals are identified, they must be translated into student-oriented, measurable objectives; Bloom's taxonomy is often used as the framework for writing objectives. Irrespective of whether formative or summative in nature, most simulated experiences are assessed according to a rubric that represents a criterion-referenced form of evaluation. Rubrics provide a clear and precise guide for both students on the essential elements of the simulation and for faculty in assessing how well students achieve those essential elements.

Rubrics should be as objective and measurable as possible. A simple rubric format that is easily adaptable to the unique features of each scenario (i.e., different courses, different learning goals, different knowledge levels among students) can be very useful. For example, when completing patient assessments, faculty might expect first-semester nursing students to meet very basic assessment competencies but would expect a senior nursing student to perform at an advanced level. In addition to the student criteria changing on the rubric, the faculty options for scoring might change. For example, if faculty let the scenario unfold according to the students' responses, then it is possible that an anticipated action may not occur; therefore, the "not applicable" category in the rubric may be very appropriate. Also, as clear and distinct as we try to be with objective criteria, often unexpected events or variations occur, making the comments section indispensable. This section is also very helpful if more than one faculty member is assessing the same student because rationale for different scores is important.

Orientation

Although it may seem basic to faculty who have worked with simulation over time, taking on the role of the nurse in any type of simulation experience can be scary and intimidating to students who are new to it. Walton, Chute, and Ball (2011) found that students felt insecure and awkward when they first started to participate in simulations. This can be partially addressed by introducing students to the scenario characters, physical or virtual environment, available supplies, and expectations. Perhaps the facilitator can walk students through the simulation first if it does not compromise the experience itself. These orientation activities can help decrease students' anxiety and even build their confidence.

Facilitation and Debriefing

An experienced facilitator who is well grounded in simulation pedagogy is needed to provide an oversight before, during, and after the experiences. This person helps ensure that the objectives are met and is able to make spur-of-the-moment modifications to ensure a successful and positive experience. Generally, the facilitator also leads the debriefing session, which is generally held immediately after the simulation so that the memories of thought processes, actions, and feelings are still fresh. The debrief should be based on a specific debriefing theoretical framework that specifically addresses the details of the specific simulation, such as the objectives, participant needs, scenario complexity, and facilitator competences (INACSL, 2016).

As mentioned in Chapter 9, the NLN (2016) provides a guide to help students think through such experiences, moving them through questions about the scenario context, content, and course. Another current debriefing framework is Promoting Excellence and Reflective Learning in Simulation (PEARLS; Eppich & Cheng, 2015). The debriefing should help participants to be reflective students and practitioners and is not complete until goals for future learning are identified. Ongoing research to guide evidence-based debriefing strategies is needed (Neill & Wotton, 2011).

High-Fidelity Patient Simulation

An HFPS experience is written as a patient situation in a clinical scenario, with students generally filling the professional role they are pursuing, but they may also fulfill other roles as called for in the scenario. The scenario specifics are determined by the learning goals. Again, a number of generic scenarios can be purchased for a variety of clinical situations, but most need at least some revision to suit a specific learning experience. HFPS can be extremely flexible in meeting objectives, so faculty should not be afraid to try new ideas.

The observer role in HFPS is gaining new interest (Bonnel & Hober, 2016). Benefits include resource effectiveness. For example, students on site might play roles in the scenario, with the experience transmitted (via live video streaming) to distance students who are the observers. In fact, there may be real value in the observer role, helping students identify concerns viewed in the scenario, articulate those issues and communicate them to others, assume accountability for their own professional responsibilities, and participate in peer review of others. Chapter 14 provides an additional discussion of this topic.

Simulated experiences can be implemented in a variety of ways. For example, in some cases faculty and students stop to discuss and plan their next steps with each change in the patient's status. This option has been used successfully, for example, in a critical care course and is very useful in helping students connect the didactic rationale to the clinical decisions they make. In addition to helping students apply critical thinking skills, with this approach faculty can choose whether to let students make mistakes. For example, students can become quite distraught if the simulated patient dies, and in some cases, faculty may want to prevent that from happening by steering students toward more appropriate actions. On the contrary, if the learning goals are focused on learning about death and dying or how to deal with poor outcomes, then it might be appropriate to let the patient "die" and help students work through their feelings.

In other classes, the simulated scenario unfolds in real time, with students taking whatever action they think the best, and the situation progressing accordingly (with the results—good or bad—depending on the student actions taken). For example, if "coded" appropriately, a simulated patient may live or die—just as real patients do, and that outcome may vary between groups of students. However, if the student gives a lethal dose of medication, the simulated patient will certainly "die."

The opportunities offered with simulations are increasing and expanding the options for using HFPSs in providing education. Simulators can be used with other teaching modalities, such as standardized (paid) patients. For example, in an interdisciplinary course focusing on intimate partner violence (IPV), a pediatric patient may be played by a pediatric HFPS who is brought to the emergency department with an asthma exacerbation. The patient's mother, who is the victim of IPV, might be played by a standardized patient. Will students focus solely on the pediatric patient, or will they also recognize the larger family issues at play in the scenario?

Electronic health records (EHRs) could also be developed for this scenario, creating a history for this patient and mother (rather than providing just the one-time glimpse into their lives represented by the scenario itself). Thus, students could look back into the medical records and find frequent emergency department visits and other events suggestive of IPV in the family. Rather than the one-moment-in-time glimpse of a patient provided by simulation alone, the EHR provides a history in which the simulated patient has a past and a context in which to manage the simulated experience.

Despite its relatively high cost, HFPS is becoming much more common in healthcare education. Breah Chambers shares her champion's experiences implementing HFPS into several programs, along with the opportunities and challenges that she has encountered, in Exhibit 12.1.

EXHIBIT 12.1

SIMULATION CHAMPION Q&A

Breah Chambers, DNP, FNP-C, APRN

1. ***How is your current position relevant to teaching with simulation technologies?*** I teach the BATI course for first-year undergraduate students. We do a lot of procedural training with task trainers and low-fidelity mannequins. I also teach and direct the simulation curriculum for the undergraduate program. We use high-fidelity, immersive simulations integrated throughout the curriculum to satisfy learning of the QSEN Institute competencies.

2. ***In what ways do you see your faculty or students benefiting from the use of simulation?*** The faculty are finally seeing the learning students get from simulations and are jumping in to help more. The students really enjoy the practice and they crave feedback. Particularly, they enjoy the interprofessional simulations.

3. ***How do you incorporate simulations, and keep students engaged, in the courses you teach or clinical experiences you supervise?*** BATI is built on psychomotor skills they practice in the laboratory. The didactic portion focuses on concepts and "why" we perform the skills/procedures. I use unfolding case studies to help them tie the procedural skills/assessments to a patient's hospital stay. During the laboratory portion of the course, students get hands-on learning, and this keeps them engaged. We ask them to practice performing every skill as if they were performing it on a real patient.

4. ***What are facilitators to incorporating simulation into your nursing education curriculum/program?*** The National Council of State Boards of Nursing (NCSBN) study (Hayden, Smiley, Alexander, Kardong-Edgren & Jeffries, 2014) suggests that 50% of clinical time could be simulation. Simulation enhances the learning of specific objectives and provides an immediate feedback related to those objectives, which they may not receive in clinical rotations. It is a way to ensure that the competencies for graduation are met in a standardized way. Simulation provides students with the ability to perform care for complex patients they may not encounter in the clinical setting and allows them to practice making the decisions rather than relying on a preceptor. The ZIEL, the University of Kansas Health System, and leadership within the university have been big influences on the drive for simulation-based education on campus.

5. ***What are the challenges of incorporating simulation into your nursing education curriculum/program?*** Simulation is resource-intense (personnel and equipment) and time-intense (development and execution), and it requires expensive equipment (mannequins and monitors). The time it takes to develop one scenario is thought to take 8 hours a week for 12 to 16 weeks. Once it is developed (using evidence-based standards), the execution of each simulation is time-consuming. Each student group of three or so is immersed in simulation and debriefing for at least 1 hour per case, with at least one technologist and one faculty for each simulation. There are also consumables (e.g., syringes, simulated medications, IV catheters, gauze), which are not reusable and cost money to replace for each simulation. Without these items, the simulation loses fidelity, and students do not get to practice their psychomotor skills.

(continued)

6. ***In what ways do you use simulations to help students learn about safety and/or quality management in clinical settings?*** We focus on safety as a concept during every class period. From the moment they walk in the room, perform hand hygiene, introduce themselves, and actively identify the patient, they are implementing safety measures. Medication administration is learned in the laboratory, and we enforce 3 MAR checks when pulling, preparing, and administering a medication. We also enforce using the safety measures such as bar-code scanners and thoroughly reading the "stop" alerts rather than clicking past them. Many simulations focus on patient safety and particularly on communication among team members.

7. ***In what ways do you have opportunity to working with interprofessional colleagues in teaching and learning with the technology?*** The medical school is revising their curriculum and integrating simulation into their first and second years, and they came to the School of Nursing for assistance with this because we have had integrated simulation in our curriculum for some time now. We decided that these students will practice together when they graduate, so why not train them together from year one? The first step was scheduling. The School of Nursing had a blank slate with the new curriculum, so we were able to schedule two simulations each semester in the first year for all 175 medical and 114 nursing students on campus. The curricular mapping of objectives has been done to both programs' competencies for accrediting agencies. The content has been cross-checked with the syllabi for each program to ensure that students have the knowledge of the disease process to adequately participate.

   In another IPE simulation, an error is forced and students conduct an RCA afterward. This simulation has evolved as the best-practice standards have emerged and as new simulation research is conducted. In the past, the students may have felt "tricked" into making an error. Now we realize the purpose of the simulation is to conduct an RCA and understand the systems issues, not allow the student to feel blame. We have limited that impact on the students by telling them that HIM students are watching and that an error may occur during the simulation. The simulation is padded heavily with system issues to ensure that the RCA is attainable for students. I am collaborating with HIM faculty to get this innovative simulation published.

8. ***What tips or advice would you like to share with the new faculty teaching with simulations?*** Understand the best-practice standards before developing or integrating simulation. Some evidence suggests that simulation can be harmful if conducted in a way that is not the best practice. Be sure to have two to three clear objectives and focus on those only. It is really easy to try and integrate 10 objectives into one simulation, but it is not as effective. Also, use validated debriefing models and practice using them regularly. This is not a skill you can perfect overnight, and it is something you have to deliberately practice on a continuous basis. The purpose of debriefing is not to critically examine the learners, but to understand their frame (e.g., why they performed an action). The only way to make a meaningful impact is to change their rationale/frame. We cannot physically see their reasoning, so we have to uncover it in debriefing. We may not completely change their frame in one simulation, but we can at least bend it.

BATI, basic assessment and therapeutic interventions; HIM, health information management; IPE, interprofessional education; MAR, medication administration record; QSEN, Quality and Safety Education for Nurses; RCA, root cause analysis; ZIEL, Zamierowski Institute for Experiential Learning.

Questions to Ask Yourself

HFPS provides a unique means to engage students in active learning experiences within the safety of a laboratory setting. Although cost once limited their availability, HFPSs are becoming increasingly available, if not in specific schools, at least regionally. However, with so many teaching options, just the availability of HFPS does not mean it is the best option. Guided by the Integrated Learning Triangle for Teaching with Technologies (Exhibit 1.3), consider the following as you think about using an HFPS experience:

1. What are the learning goals? Will a simulated experience help students achieve those goals?
2. What other teaching options are available that could also help students achieve the learning goals?
3. Which of the teaching options is the best fit? For example, if two options are considered equally effective in meeting the learning goals, the best fit is likely the least expensive, less time-consuming option. HFPSs are very expensive, as are their repairs, so why risk overuse and damage to the simulator if a less-expensive option is also available?
4. What support do you have for using the HFPS? Although one faculty member may be sufficient to oversee the scenario, at the very least an additional staff/faculty member needs to be available to program and run the simulator. Also, is the simulator available when needed, or is it already booked for another class?
5. How will you achieve the learning goals if something prevents the HFPS from operating on a scheduled day? What other options are there for presenting this material as a backup plan?

If you need additional resources and support, the NLN offers an online SIRC. This is an excellent resource for faculty both new to and experienced with HFPS. Further resources in developing and guiding simulations are also being published in journals and texts, including frameworks such as those provided by Jeffries (2012) and Nehring and Lashley (2009). Also, an abstract of an evidence-based review, "Faculty Orientation to Learning Simulation," is shared in Exhibit 12.2. This systematic review provides direction for developing faculty orientation programs for simulation.

EXHIBIT 12.2

EVIDENCE-BASED REVIEW ABSTRACT: FACULTY ORIENTATION TO LEARNING SIMULATION

Compiled by Christine L. Hober, PhD, RN-BC, CNE

The following summary provides a graduate student's experience conducting an evidence-based review on the topic of faculty orientation to the use of simulation.

Leaders in nursing education are implementing simulation for the interactive, collaborative, time-orientated experiential learning milieu that better prepares students for the real world of nursing. Simulation is known to engage the student in the scholarship of learning and teaching while providing direction for clinical training using the seven

(continued)

principles of best practice as discussed by Chickering and Gamson (1987). While simulation is a learning tool that requires technological knowledge and aptitude, research indicates that faculty have limited technological competence.

This issue, coupled with nursing faculty shortages and national budgetary concerns, creates surmountable barriers to implementing simulation technology in practicum and theoretical venues. One possible solution is to facilitate the transition of faculty into simulation technology through structured orientation programs. This abstract synthesizes the literature for faculty orientation to infuse simulation into nursing curricula. Findings from the systematic literature review reveal that faculty simulation orientation programs need to be sustained over a period of time, be incorporated into faculty development plans, foster an open and invigorating informatics environment, connect accessible simulation mentors with faculty, and have institutional support.

The research findings go on to show that informatic competencies must be infused into nursing curricula and faculty development plans to expand a nursing community of practice for prudent informatics technologies. This process can be augmented using a change model and a phased approach to bridge the gap of simulation technology with faculty development and curriculum innovations (Jeffries, 2008).

The essential factors of facilitating faculty ownership of simulation focus on provision of standardized materials easily accessible to faculty in a timely manner, ample time to train and retrain faculty, simulation design through integration teams, and ongoing simulation development and evaluation activities for faculty and students. Insightful research and lessons learned stress the applicability of simulation permeation using faculty expertise.

Ultimately, nursing educators will be taking a step toward the best practices in nursing education while working toward high-quality patient care for the next generation of professional nurses by implementing simulation competence. Simulation provides an opportunity for nurse educators to redesign educational programs to meet the needs of today's students.

Virtual Worlds

Although virtual serious games provide many options similar to simulation, it offers different strengths and weaknesses. For example, the simulated experience offers more lifelike interactions, so if interpersonal skills are included in the expected outcomes, virtual world gaming may not be the best option available. However, if learning outcomes include learning about connecting patients with community resources, for example, then gaming may provide the better option. Gaming also offers the potential for synchronous and asynchronous interactions, and this convenience is often very attractive to students. Virtual worlds also tend to be far less expensive because they do not carry the high price tag and maintenance of HFPSs and have much greater accessibility because a good computer is the only required equipment (Verkuyl et al., 2017).

As described earlier, students play themselves in the electronic virtual world as an avatar, and through this avatar, their thoughts, decisions, and actions are expressed in the virtual world. Second Life provides one gaming option in which virtual worlds, such as hospitals or community clinics, can be created and in which the students can practice clinical and critical thinking skills. The roles students play and the nature and unfolding of the game itself can vary widely. Like HFPS, electronic gaming can be extremely flexible in meeting objectives, so do not be afraid to try new ideas.

Shadow Health is a virtual simulation with laboratories where increasing clinical hours are completed (refer to Online Resources for Further Learning). Studies find that virtual gaming combined with hands-on simulation positively affects students' knowledge, self-efficacy, and learning satisfaction and is recommended as the best teaching and learning practice (Verkuyl et al., 2017).

Resources specific to virtual world gaming are available to guide your work. Best practices for game-based learning (McDaniel, 2009) provide direction. McDaniel's suggestions are as follows: Take advantage of resources, do not be overly prescriptive, focus on the learning rather than the technology, provide preparation for the game and debriefing, encourage interdisciplinarity, and test and revise the game often.

Questions to Ask Yourself

As with HFPSs, just because gaming is available does not mean it is the best option. Guided by the Integrated Learning Triangle for Teaching With Technologies (Exhibit 1.3), ask yourself the same questions when trying to decide if gaming is the best teaching approach in a given situation:

1. What are the learning goals? Will a gaming experience help students achieve those goals?
2. What other teaching options are available that could also help students achieve the learning goals?
3. Which of the teaching options is the best fit? For example, if you are teaching cultural competence, students might be very engaged in a new, virtual culture that is different from any other culture they have ever experienced (if the faculty is very creative and develops a setting with entirely new creatures and customs and language). This option, however, requires a great deal of preparation time and effort, and although it may teach valuable lessons, the actual customs learned will not have any real-world application because faculty made the world up. Another option for teaching the content might be to have a service learning project in which students go to a community center and care for elderly clients of a particular ethnic background. This experience might serve the same purpose of teaching valuable lessons about cultural competence, as well as actual customs that would have real-world applicability, without using gaming at all.
4. How will you achieve the learning goals if something prevents you and the students from logging into the virtual space on a particular day? What other options are there for presenting this material as a backup plan?

CLINICAL EDUCATION AND HEALTH PROFESSIONS IMPLICATIONS

Because of its ability to teach application of critical thinking skills while still addressing the issue of patient safety, simulation is an excellent method for teaching the Quality and Safety Education for Nurses Institute (QSEN; 2017) and Interprofessional Education Collaborative (IPEC; 2016) clinical competencies. Simulated and gaming experiences provide the same advantages to healthcare providers who need to demonstrate new or ongoing proficiency on select clinical knowledge and skills as they do to students. Many hospitals, for example, require that staff recertify on cardiopulmonary resuscitation (CPR) and demonstrate competency in other skills on a regular basis. Similarly, education/demonstration experiences are required of staff as procedures and equipment are updated; simulated experiences may be an appropriate and efficient mechanism for teaching and evaluating mastery of that knowledge and skills.

INTEGRATED LEARNING TRIANGLE FOR TEACHING WITH TECHNOLOGIES

Although falling most directly in the teaching and learning activities and feedback/assessment categories, the content about simulation and gaming in this chapter involves the entire Triangle of Integrated Learning for Teaching With Technologies. Both are supported by educational theories and best practices. For example, through HFPS or Second Life, students actively participate in creating their own knowledge for immediate application, consistent with adult learning theory and constructivism.

The teaching and learning activities and feedback/assessment activities are guided most directly by learning goals and objectives, so that connection is strong. For example, if the learning goal is CPR and the lower-technology option is adequate to achieve the learning goal, then it may well be the better option because it does not require the greater sophistication and delicacy of the more expensive HFPS to achieve the same goal.

Similarly, the teaching and learning and feedback/assessment options discussed in this chapter depend directly on situational factors that include logistics, resources, and context. If your school or clinical site does not own or have access to an HFPS, then that is not an option. If you do not have a person with gaming expertise who also has the time and interest to work with you, then gaming may not be a good option. Consider the available resources in terms of personnel, expertise, expense, time, and fit when deciding what technologies should be used in a given situation.

You too are part of the situational factors. In addition to newly emerging technologies, both HFPS and virtual world gaming are experiencing constant upgrades, so the literature and the options change rapidly. Your commitment to lifelong learning will determine, in part, your willingness to try new teaching options, as well as your ability to use it effectively to contribute to evidence-based best practices. Faculty is required to be aware of their pivotal role in affecting the situational context.

SUMMARY

Simulation offers a new and exciting method for teaching healthcare professionals. Advantages include immersion in the real, though virtual, world; active learning; safety; and effectiveness. However, faculty are required to use excellent critical thinking skills to determine which simulated experiences are the best for any given situation. Faculty also need to keep up as the best practices are identified and revised, especially regarding topics such as rubrics, orientation, and debriefing strategies.

ENDING REFLECTIONS FOR YOUR LEARNING NOTEBOOK

1. What is the most important content that you learned in this chapter?
2. What are your plans for using the information provided in this chapter in your future teaching endeavors?
3. What are your further learning goals?

GUIDELINES FOR TEACHING AND LEARNING WITH TECHNOLOGIES

Quick Teaching Tips

1. In a debriefing, be sure to include all students (with eye contact. by name, or both) equally if there are more students participating in the debriefing than participated in an actual scenario or game.
2. Consider using standardized case studies for simulation or gaming, especially if you are new to that technology. Do not hesitate to tailor the standardized case to your specific learning objectives.
3. Remember quality-improvement approaches. As with most teaching activities, simulated or gaming experiences generally improve as they are continually revised and reimplemented in subsequent semesters.

Questions for Further Reflection

1. In many ways, simulations and gaming are merely extensions of the traditional case study. In what ways are the three similar and in what ways are they different?
2. Think of the topics that you already teach, or plan to teach in the future. Do any lend themselves to simulation and/or gaming? On what rationale did you base your answers?

Learning Activity: Teaching Range of Motion

The purpose of this activity is to explore different options for using simulation to teach a long-standing clinical skill

1. You have been assigned to teach the content on range of motion (ROM) to students. Consider and discuss the following:
   a. What would your learning goals be for students?
   b. What would a ROM learning experience look like on a HFPS (describe the scenario, student roles, rubrics)?
   c. What would a ROM learning experience look like in Second Life (describe the virtual world, student roles, rubrics)?
   d. What other teaching methods could be used to teach the content?
   e. What aspects of the learning experience would you consider when deciding on the teaching method you would use to teach the ROM content?
   f. How would your activities change if you were evaluating students' ROM competency rather than teaching the ROM content?

Online Resources for Further Learning

- Shadow Health. The QSEN Institute has partnered with Shadow Health to infuse QSEN competencies into Digital Clinical Healthcare Experiences for undergraduate and graduate students. shadowhealth .com
- NLN, SIRC. This site offers faculty a variety of online opportunities for learning about integrating simulation into nursing curricula. sirc.nln .org
- INACSL. This site has tips for managing a simulation center, as well as links to numerous resource centers. inacsl.org

REFERENCES

Beaubien, J. M., & Baker, D. P. (2004). The use of simulation for training teamwork skills in health care: How low can you go? *Quality and Safety in Health Care*, *13*(Suppl. 1), i51–i56. doi:10.1136/qhc.13. suppl_1.i51. Retrieved from http://qshc.bmj.com/cgi/content/abstract/13/suppl_1/i51

Bonnel, W., & Hober, C. (2016). Optimizing the reflective observer role in high-fidelity patient simulation. *Journal of Nursing Education*, *55*(6), 353–356. doi:10.3928/01484834-20160516-10

Chickering, A. W., & Gamson, Z. F. (1987). Seven principles for good practice in undergraduate education. Retrieved from https://files.eric.ed.gov/fulltext/ED282491.pdf

Eppich, W., & Cheng, A. (2015). Promoting Excellence and Reflective Learning in Simulation (PEARLS): Development and rationale for a blended approach to health care simulation debriefing. *Simulation in Healthcare*, *10*(2), 106–115. doi:10.1097/SIH.0000000000000072

Hayden, J. K., Smiley, R. A., Alexander, M., Kardong-Edgren, S., & Jeffries, P. R. (2014). The NCSBN national simulation study: A longitudinal, randomized, controlled study replacing clinical hours with simulation in prelicensure nursing education. *Journal of Nursing Regulation*, *5*(2), C1–S64.

International Nursing Association for Clinical Simulation and Learning. (2016). INACSL standards of best practice: Simulation. Retrieved from https://www.inacsl.org/i4a/pages/index.cfm?pageid=3407

Interprofessional Education Collaborative. (2016). *Core competencies for interprofessional collaborative practice: 2016 update*. Washington, DC: Author.

Jeffries, P. R. (2008). Getting in S.T.E.P. with simulations: Simulations take educator preparation. *Nursing Education Perspectives, 29*(2), 70–73. doi:10.1097/00024776-200803000-00006

Jeffries, P. R. (2012). *Simulation in nursing education: From conceptualization to evaluation* (2nd ed.). New York, NY: National League for Nursing.

McDaniel, R. (2009). Best practices for integrating game-based learning into online teaching. Retrieved from http://jolt.merlot.org/vol5no2/mcdaniel_0609.htm

National League for Nursing. (2016). Critical Conversations: The NLN guide for teaching thinking. Retrieved from http://www.nln.org/search?query=critical%20conversations

Nehring, W., & Lashley, F. (2009). *High-fidelity patient simulation in nursing education*. Boston, MA: Jones & Bartlett.

Neill, M. A., & Wotton, K. (2011). High fidelity simulation debriefing in nursing education: A literature review. Retrieved from http://www.nursingsimulation.org/article/S1876-1399(11)00026-0/pdf

Quality and Safety Education for Nurses Institute. (2017). QSEN competencies. Retrieved from http://qsen.org/competencies

Verkuyl, M., Romaniuk, D., Atack, L., & Mastrilli, P. (2017). Virtual gaming simulation for nursing education: An experiment. *Clinical Simulation in Nursing, 13*, 238–244. doi:10.1016/j.ecns.2017.02.004

Walton, J., Chute, E., & Ball, L. (2011). Negotiating the role of the professional nurse. Retrieved from http://www.professionalnursing.org/article/S8755-7223(11)00042-1/fulltext

Informatics: Teaching Clinical Data Management for Populations and Systems Health

CHAPTER GOAL

Gain teaching and learning strategies to help students think critically and work responsibly with data and information systems.

BEGINNING REFLECTION

1. What are your experiences guiding students in learning about clinical data management and health information systems?
2. What further goals will help you and your students stay current with data management?

Overheard: *What is this nursing informatics all about? I'm not even sure I know what that means.*

Informatics and technologies are changing the face of healthcare. Informatics and technology provide opportunity to enhance communication, support nursing care processes, and lead to outcome analysis (National League for Nursing [NLN], 2015). Nursing students are preparing for a future in which concepts of data management will be pervasive throughout clinical care. Students will be using technologies to gather and use data in assessing, planning, and evaluating individuals. Teaching and learning broad concepts of data management in healthcare are central to safe, quality patient care. Helping students understand the basics of data collection and data management with a variety of patients, populations, and purposes is a key faculty role.

Pedagogy guides faculty in setting up lesson plans and clinical assignments to help students develop a skill set in data management. Guided by educational theories and best evidence, faculty can develop activities and assignments that promote ongoing student knowledge gain, with data management as the central concept. Helping students learn to promote safe, efficient patient care using data management tools is an important faculty goal (American Association of Colleges of Nursing [AACN], 2008). Students learn decision making and critical thinking as part of informatics (McGonigle & Mastrian, 2017).

This chapter focuses on data management in clinical settings, with information systems such as electronic health records (EHRs) to help students learn to provide quality care and promote patient safety. Concepts to be discussed related to information management and information systems include the importance of this topic, opportunities for teaching and learning with EHRs, varied teaching and learning opportunities specific to informatics, and broad curricular issues in nursing education.

IMPORTANCE OF TEACHING INFORMATION MANAGEMENT AND INFORMATION SYSTEMS

Data for decision making incorporate all aspects of healthcare. Informatics combines nursing science, information science, and computer science (McGonigle & Mastrian, 2017). Historically, clinical data have been handwritten on charts, with information organized manually. The advent of computers and health information programs now provides opportunities for rapidly collecting and organizing even very large data sets. Now computers help clinicians assess and problem solve not only for an individual but also for large populations.

With the rapid advance of informatics in healthcare, a variety of professional organizations have confirmed the need for students to rapidly learn about informatics. These organizations also provide resources that can be used to assist and extend student learning (see Exhibit 13.1).

EXHIBIT 13.1

EXAMPLES OF ORGANIZATIONS SUPPORTING INFORMATICS EDUCATION

Understanding concepts of informatics and data management has been deemed critical by a variety of respected organizations. Sample organizations supporting integrating of informatics and providing resources include the following:

- The NLN has published a position paper focusing on faculty preparation, "Preparing the Next Generation of Nurses to Practice in a Technology-Rich Environment: An Informatics Agenda": www.nln.org/aboutnln/PositionStatements/index.htm
- The ANA has recognized informatics as a specialty for many years, maintaining the "Nursing Informatics: Scope and Standards of Practice" document. This text is available through Nursing World books.
- AACN incorporates informatics competencies in its "Baccalaureate Essentials" document, discussing specific tools, as well as the process of using informatics tools to promote safe, quality care: www.aacn.nche.edu/Education/bacessn.htm

(continued)

- The IOM (2003) "Health Professions Educator Report: A Bridge to Quality," reports, emphasizes the need to educate the health professions in informatics: www.nap .edu/catalog/10681/health-professions-education-a-bridge-to-quality
- The TIGER Initiative provides leadership on promoting informatics competencies in nursing programs, as well as developing technology and informatics best practices for health professions: www.himss.org/tiger-initiative-reports
- The QSEN initiative, funded by The Robert Wood Johnson Foundation, provides a repository for classroom assignments with relevance to several broad areas of health professions education: www.qsen.org
- HIMSS. This not-for-profit U.S. organization aims to promote better understanding of healthcare information and management systems: www.himss.org/ASP/index.asp

AACN, American Association of Colleges of Nursing; ANA, American Nurses Association; HIMSS, Healthcare Information and Management Systems Society; IOM, Institute of Medicine; NLN, National League for Nursing; TIGER, Technology Informatics Guiding Educational Reform; QSEN, Quality and Safety Education for Nurses.

As a general guide, we want students to understand the benefits that information management and electronic information systems provide to a variety of entities, including patients, healthcare professionals, consumers, payers, and healthcare systems. Coiera (2015) summarized research supporting the following benefits to electronic information systems:

- ***Documentation for safe practice.*** Preventing errors in patient care is a major concern, including not only clarity of written information, but also enhanced communication among all responsible professionals.
- ***Quality improvement***. Providing quality care is enhanced by reflecting on information about practice. Electronic records provide the opportunity for quality improvement, including data feedback mechanisms.
- ***Patient self-care***. Patients ideally have opportunities for gaining their own electronic personal records that will be available wherever they seek healthcare; this provides care continuity and safety in clinical care.
- ***Team communication***. Information systems (including electronic order entry, record keeping, and sharing of information between appropriate departments such as laboratories and pharmacies) promote team communication.
- ***Decision support***. Rather than replacing decision making, electronic systems provide opportunities to monitor and support nurses' clinical decision making. Electronic systems serve as a type of tutorial role for health professionals.
- ***Monitoring***. Information systems provide opportunities for monitoring patient data and patient trends over time.

Information management consists of a number of related concepts. Information literacy and evidence-based practice, as discussed in earlier chapters, are intertwined with this topic. Computer literacy serves as just one component of informatics.

TEACHING AND LEARNING CRITICAL THINKING WITH ELECTRONIC HEALTH RECORDS AND DATA SETS

Information management systems can help students learn to organize data. Because most patients present with multiple, diverse symptoms, grouping patient data into patterns helps students make sense of it. Informatics incorporates the complexity of patterns and helps students organize or make sense of multiple pieces of data. For example, a patient's leg edema, shortness of breath, and weight gain are isolated facts for a new assessor. Electronic assessment forms support students' critical thinking skills to bring these data bits together as a pattern consistent with congestive heart failure. Students learn as individual patient data bits become patterns of information and then knowledge. Students learn about data being used in the following ways:

- To group data to first provide information and then to provide knowledge (whether for individual patients or large population groups)
- To follow outcome-based practice via automated clinical pathways with databases to study care processes and outcomes
- To enhance clinical outcomes by decreasing errors, managing knowledge and information, making evidence-based decisions, and improving communication (Institute of Medicine [IOM], 2001)

Electronic Health Record as Learning Tool

Faculty use EHRs to teach students judgment and information processing for both individual patients and patient populations. The EHR is a legal record created in hospitals and ambulatory environments that serves as the central source of patient data (Healthcare Information and Management Systems Society [HIMSS], n.d.). Central elements of these tools specific to direct patient care include standardized forms with key terms and definitions that promote consistency in data collection.

EHRs have multiple core functions, including clinical documentation and order entry, clinical messaging, result reporting, data repository, and decision support (Hebda & Czar, 2014). The EHR also brings together information from a variety of departments, such as test results from laboratories and current medications from pharmacies. Information systems support clinical care delivery. They facilitate and transform data collection and use. With its standardized terminology and templates, it serves as an example of an electronic information management system and data set for student learning. Students gain in learning the following:

- Computers serve as tools for aggregating patient assessment data and then organizing those data to identify a problem and develop a plan for patient care.

- Electronic records provide a type of electronic worksheet for gathering data and helping clarify and combine random facts to provide synthesized information.
- Students learn to think critically and manage information for patient problem solving and care planning using these tools.
- Students assess, record, and review patient data in practicing these skills.
- Students gain understanding of how separate pieces of data from assessments all come together for problem clarification and decision making.
- Information systems help collect and organize the data to help healthcare providers identify problems more efficiently for individual patients (as well as larger populations).

EHRs, important tools for faculty work with students, not only bring benefits, but also select challenges, in providing teaching and learning opportunities. An experienced educator and researcher, Dr. Helene Winstanley shares her champion experiences related to moving EHRs into the curriculum in Exhibit 13.2. She provides interesting discussion of sample challenges and strategies faculty have shared with her in her research.

EXHIBIT 13.2

ELECTRONIC HEALTH RECORDS CHAMPION Q & A

Helene Winstanley, PhD, RN, ANP-C, CCRN-K

1. ***What is your current position? What formal or informal education or training have you had in your current position?*** I am currently a Professor of Nursing at Suffolk County Community College in New York. I have used EHRS for more than 10 years as an RN, NP, and nurse educator/clinical instructor. As part of my PhD coursework in Nursing, I completed a Health Professions Educator Certificate, which included content in teaching with technologies. Previous relevant experiences included a Biomedical Informatics Course Fellow at a marine biological laboratory sponsored by the National Library of Medicine (2011) and a faculty-development program as a Health Information Technology Scholar sponsored in part by the NLN (2010).

   As a clinical instructor and a practicing RN, I was initially intrigued by the effects of transitioning to EHRS on nurses and nurse–patient relationships. I realized that the integration of EHRS in our healthcare facilities was presenting significant challenges for my nursing program, such as restricted access to the EHRS and limited opportunities to document or review records. On campus, faculty face challenges that include acquiring an EHRS to meet teaching needs and integrating EHRS and informatics into the curriculum. These experiences led me to wonder whether this was affecting other programs, especially other associate degree nursing programs, so my dissertation research explored the experiences, perspectives, challenges, and teaching strategies of associate degree nursing faculty related to teaching students to use EHRS (Winstanley, 2017).

2. ***What are some of the issues you find related to EHRS and schools of nursing? What issues exist specific to classrooms? To the clinical setting? For continuity from classroom to***

(continued)

clinical? The most striking concern is the variation in EHRS use across schools of nursing. Based on both anecdotal reports and the literature, many faculty are working to increase the accessibility and integration of EHRS in their prelicensure programs (Winstanley, 2017). A wide range of factors affect EHRS adoption and implementation in a program, including curricular integration, faculty acceptance/approval and development, cost and ongoing maintenance of an academic EHRS product, usability and support of the product, and ability to update the product. For many programs, clinical practice access and use area depended on their clinical partners. Some academic products allow for documentation of clinical assignments, but cautions about maintaining privacy must be addressed. Some programs benefit from the ability to use the same EHRS in both the classroom and clinical sites, improving continuity and lessening the challenge of teaching across EHRS platforms.

3. *What are key points that nurse educator students would need to understand related to EHRS and teaching and learning issues in nursing programs (i.e., why this is important to understand)?* EHRS use is increasingly integrated into practicing nurses' workflow for routine tasks. Accordingly, nursing students need to learn how to navigate the EHRS, use it to access relevant information, and document appropriately (Winstanley, 2017). To prepare students for practice, faculty seek opportunities for students to progressively use the EHRS and integrate it into their developing nursing practice. Building time on task, repetition, and depth of understanding of EHRS through active learning strategies will improve expertise.

4. *What are select challenges of using EHRS assignments to engage individuals? What recommendations are there for ongoing needs/work?* As with any technology, there are inherent challenges associated with access to computers and software for students. Computer competencies among students may vary; not all students are digital natives, and many lack the necessary skills to navigate the EHRS. Access to EHRS or academic EHRS may not extend beyond the clinical or classroom setting, making it difficult for students to practice or complete homework assignments. Legal issues, especially those affecting patient confidentiality and information security, require special attention. The latter includes concerns for error recognition and mitigation to prevent any impact to patients (Winstanley, 2017).

5. *What are select facilitators for incorporating the use of EHRS to engage individuals on select topics? What are some of the positive things faculty report that they are doing related to EHRS?* Faculty leverage the setting for opportunities to teach EHRS use (Winstanley, 2017). Recommendations focus on increasing the use of academic EHRS designed to optimize student learning and practice time while facilitating faculty use and effectiveness. Integrating EHRS use and informatics concepts with nursing practice and role playing during all nonclinical classes prepares students to use EHRS more efficiently during clinical classes (and it is hoped, into professional practice). Deliberately including progressive EHRS use in the curricula may enhance student expertise. Having a user-friendly academic EHRS and individual access to the EHRS in clinical settings are significant facilitators. Some faculty take advantage of an academic EHRS to project excerpts or screen shots into the classroom as they lectured or present a case study, mimicking clinical practice.

The nursing laboratory is used to introduce the EHRS and build rudimentary skills. Some are integrating EHRS use, most often documentation, into simulation activities, despite concerns about time constraints. In clinical settings, faculty use demonstration, observation, and direct experience to maximize students' experiences with EHRS. When available, clinical decision support tools are used for background information and for support of evidence-based practice. Faculty described using the EHRS to help students connect information in the EHRS with direct patient care and professional nursing behaviors.

(continued)

6. **What advice would you like to share with new or future nurse educators about what you have learned regarding the integration of EHRS into nursing programs?** Take advantage of coursework and continuing education courses in informatics, population health, and teaching with technologies because they would be most helpful. Faculty participants of my study offered advice for faculty new to teaching about EHRS (Winstanley, 2017). Training for specific EHRS in your teaching practice will improve proficiency. Try to spend time learning the EHRS and academic EHRS and work with staff and/or the super-users. Allow for time to learn and get comfortable with the systems before teaching students. Assess clinical partners' opportunities for students to use their EHRS, noting any rules or limitations to access or use. There is a significant need for faculty with expertise in teaching and using EHRS.

7. **What resources will be useful to guide new faculty in this area?** As noted, graduate coursework and continuing education courses in informatics, population health, and teaching with technologies would be most helpful. Training for specific EHRS in teaching practice will improve proficiency. Moreover, there are online resources available. Sample resources include: ONC (www.healthit.gov) and the QSEN Institute (http://qsen.org).

EHRS, Electronic Health Record Systems; NLN, National League for Nursing; ONC, Office of the National Coordinator for Health Information Technology; QSEN, Quality and Safety Education for Nurses.

Winstanley, H. D. (2017). *A qualitative descriptive study exploring associate degree nursing faculty's experiences teaching electronic health record systems use* (Doctoral dissertation). University of Kansas Medical Center, Kansas City, KS.

Standardized Electronic Assessment Forms

EHRs provide a type of standardized assessment form. Students gain a useful resource as they learn the benefits of the standardized assessment forms that EHRs provide. In teaching about EHRs, it is important that students think about the way that a particular EHR system is set up in terms of embedded questions and definitions in the electronic assessment forms. They need to understand that the EHRs are more than just checking boxes on the computer screen. In addition to gaining a baseline of assessment data on individual patients, these tools provide the following:

- A descriptive summary report of individual patients.
- Data for comparisons over time. Students learn that this information also helps compare patient progress over time. Although providers have monitored patients' status over time, often because of various healthcare system issues, access to clear comparison data for tracking patient progress was lacking.
- Reminder cues for thorough assessments. These tools provide cues that help students recall and avoid missing critical assessment questions. For example, when completing an assessment on a preoperative patient, cues provide reminders to question whether a patient has a history of sleep apnea or has stopped specific medications, which are critical history questions. These EHR reminders also assist students in recording clear, concise, and complete information.

- Grouping of multiple individual's data. Students learn that this information can help describe populations and then make comparisons across patient populations. For a beginning assignment in the classroom, case examples of different patient data collected on standardized formats might be grouped and discussed.
- Documentation of characteristics of both the individual patient and broader populations. Benefits to healthcare organizations exist in tracking selected data. For example, the Long Term Care Minimum Data Set (MDS), a comprehensive system for electronic data management in long-term care, uses assessment information systems for tracking selected variables such as patient nutrition.

Although students typically see the implications of data use for individual patients, EHR assignments can help them extend this learning to populations. They begin to consider the benefits of understanding population data and the potential impact on care of groups of patients by using standardized electronic data that compare, for example, data on their patient population with diabetes.

Electronic Health Records as Tools for Care Planning and Evaluation

Standardized plans of care and resources for monitoring clinical pathways/outcomes are integral to the EHR and provide important student learning tools. Once patient problems have been identified, decision-support technologies can generate plans of care from evidence-based standards and protocols. Students then use critical thinking in confirming the appropriateness of the generated plan for a specified patient. As plans are implemented, information systems allow further monitoring of patients' progress. Consistency with clinical pathways and anticipated outcomes can be monitored. A common example of clinical pathways is use of core measures by hospitals on selected diagnoses to document quality care outcomes (The Joint Commission, 2017). Faculty might share a case example of a core measure such as acute myocardial infarction to help students see the importance of these pathways.

Although clinical pathways provide broad, general patient care direction, clinicians' critical thinking is key in applying judgment to the patient's specific context. Additional critical thinking opportunities emerge for students when they care for patients with clinical problems that have not yet been well researched and developed into evidence-based protocols. As noted by McGonigle and Mastrian (2017), the whole point of information management is to support good decision making, the goal we have for our students.

VARIED TEACHING AND LEARNING OPPORTUNITIES WITH ELECTRONIC INFORMATION SYSTEMS

Just as faculty use data from student and academic affairs offices to better understand student population characteristics and needs, students can be helped to better understand the use of data for documenting patient characteristics and care needs. Learning about clinical data sets helps students gain tools that have broad implications for patient care quality and safety. Assignments can be developed that help students relate or connect data specific to their individual patients to broader populations. Students can learn the importance of monitoring population variables to help document outcomes in their clinical units or agencies. Teaching quality improvement and population health provide important opportunities with the EHR. A sample assignment could relate to traditional community health needs assessment and recording of population data for comparisons across regional, state, and national databases.

Teaching Continuous Quality Improvement

Information systems are important in helping students think about projects such as quality improvement. EHRs allow not only easy access to collected data for individual patients in hospitals and community healthcare settings, but also opportunity to generate questions and compile data for specific populations. In the hospital, an example of this quality-improvement approach would include monitoring and studying information about variables related to clinical unit falls and adverse clinical events. Although data sets are tools that nurses have used for years, their use has been limited because of the time-consuming manual manipulation of data. Stacks of paper copies, initially recorded a unit's history of patient falls over a specified time. These might later be collated, but information analysis was at a distant point in time. Information management systems change this dynamic, allowing information to be compiled rapidly. As faculty, we can now help students use information management systems that provide more efficiency in quality-assurance processes and lead to better, safer care for patients. Further discussion of quality improvement concepts is provided in Chapter 9.

Teaching Population and Public Health With Information Technologies

Many teaching and learning opportunities exist to engage students in documenting the populations they are caring for in clinical settings or public health arenas. For example, information technologies such as Typhon are not new for student data reporting, but they provide a valuable tool to help students tell the story of their practice populations. As students seek to learn primary care of individuals they often neglect opportunities to gain a populations perspective of their practice. The Reflective Reports assignment can help students become accountable for their population practice and gain needed portfolio documents. The experiential Reflective Reports assignment, enhancing the traditional clinical log, helps students describe their practice, identify practice needs, make practice change recommendations, and identify topics for future clinical projects/study. The assignment includes the addition of reflective questions to electronic graphic reports of clinical logs, helping students address the "so what and what next" related to their practice populations. An important step in advocating for and leading practice change, it can help them identify practice needs,

EXHIBIT 13.3

REFLECTIVE POPULATION REPORTS

The Reflective Reports assignment, adding to the traditional student electronic logs, includes the addition of reflective questions to electronic graphic reports to help students add the "what, so what, and what next?" to their clinical logs. Purpose: Describe the nurse practitioner student assignment, Reflective Reports, including the assignment process and evaluation. Reflective Reports help students reflect on electronic reports such as Typhon to learn clinical population perspectives. Nurse practitioner core competencies (NONPF, 2017) emphasize the value of engaging students to integrate technology, communicate practice knowledge, and consider practice change needs to improve practice and practice knowledge. Evaluative Methods: A systems model of structure/process/outcome guides the evaluative project. Retrospective assignment review, evaluative data, and sample products from three semesters indicated that students valued this assignment with sample reflective comments: "I had no idea I was seeing so many Medicaid pts" and "I was surprised by the actual ages and diagnoses that I was seeing most often." Emphasizing reflective questions with electronic graphic reports adds practice value and provides important products for students' future work, including documented need for future clinical projects, reports for their portfolios and future credentialing needs, and comfort with electronic reports to help name and describe their future population practices.

recommendations, and topics for future study. An example of the Reflective Population Report assignment is provided in Exhibit 13.3.

Informatics tools can be used to support public health. Examples that include community health risk assessment (tools for knowledge acquisition, monitoring of disease outbreaks/epidemiology, and agency support); knowledge for health disaster planning and preparation, support of communication, and dissemination to a population; and use of feedback to promote readiness and improve responses (McGonigle & Mastrian, 2017). Other assignments could focus on gaining familiarity with local (and regional or national) public health informatics networks and could include examples of public health disease surveillance and outbreak management.

Useful resources with a web presence for assignments such as virtual tours and teaching public health topics include the following:

- Centers for Disease Control and Prevention (CDC)
- Healthy People 2020
- American Public Health Association
- Public Health Informatics (one of the three centers within the CDC)
- Center for Public Health Informatics

Although nursing educators may not be experts in all public health arenas, a population and public health focus is important to all. Networking with informatics nurse clinicians to gain speakers for classes and arrange student clinical experiences on these topics extends teaching, learning, and practice opportunities.

CURRICULAR ISSUES FOR FURTHER THOUGHT

Nursing informatics (NI) is a curricular issue. Informatics concepts and definitions are evolving, and faculty do not always understand or agree on descriptors. Expanded emphasis for faculty discussions about NI and curriculum includes topics such as the following:

- Data and technologies for problem solving. What type of assignments count?
- Opportunities to engage students in using EHR data to document care processes and outcomes.
- Occasions to help students use technologies in considering healthcare systems and populations, as well as leadership and policy issues.
- Basic introduction to big data, using large national data sets such as the National Database of Nursing Quality Indicators (NDNQI).
- Determine if specific national organization competencies are addressed in the curriculum and to what extent.

With the central role of informatics in healthcare, informatics becomes a curricular issue. Faculty need to consider how best to integrate NI into their curriculum and appreciate that one class session on informatics is insufficient if further relevant content is not integrated across the curriculum. Informatics competencies need to be implemented in all levels of nursing education consistent with recommendations from diverse professional organizations, as summarized by Clancy (2015). Diverse competencies have been proposed for health professionals. Many of these competencies take a novice to advanced practitioner approach. They advance beyond basic computer competencies to incorporate competencies related to data, data impact, data privacy/security, and data systems.

In addition, team roles and collaboration are important considerations with healthcare information systems. These tools are not used in isolation. Students need to know about contributing to the development of EHR systems and being a part of the team. Systems theory states that all components of a system are interactive, so all team members need to be well versed in these tools—including the standardized language and type of data they provide. The AACN (2008) indicates that students need to be aware of their roles as team members, which includes attention to best workflow design in EHR systems. Students can learn the concept of participating as team members and advocate for designs that are both effective and efficient in patient care. In particular, these tools have potential to enhance team communication about patient care among diverse providers and across disciplines.

Informatics Variability Across Populations and Healthcare Settings

EHRs are still evolving and vary by clinical sites. Many clinical sites still use unique systems, standards, and practices, with limited communication across settings beyond the immediate practice. In the past, the challenges in tracking documentation in healthcare were referred to as a black hole, indicating the need for further attention to this challenge. Many issues exist around inconsistencies and cumbersome programs as healthcare systems seek to gain EHRs. If there are different systems in different settings students will be working in, they need to understand the general concepts of EHRs and then be prepared to adapt to alternate formats. Faculty have described this as an ongoing concern (Winstanley, 2017).

The newness and ongoing changes and updates to EHR systems can present challenges to keeping students competent. Staff nurses themselves are often challenged to gain data management expertise in new or updated systems in their clinical agencies. As noted, the challenges related to EHRs, and ideas for faculty to consider are described by EHRs champion Helene Winstanley in Exhibit 13.2.

Ethical and Legal Issues

A variety of ethical issues related to data management exist that students need to know. Issues related to data management include the privacy rule and the Health Insurance Portability and Accountability Act (HIPAA). The privacy rule or standards for the privacy of individually identifiable health information were issued to implement the requirements of the HIPAA (U.S. Department of Health and Human Services, 2003). The rule provides national standards regarding the disclosure of health information, seeking a balance between protecting individual's privacy and the flow of information needed to provide quality care. AACN (2008) makes clear that patient rights and ownership of the EHR are topics to be considered in nursing classrooms. Keeping information safe and private is the theme.

ACADEMIC ELECTRONIC HEALTH RECORDS IN THE CLASSROOM

Opportunities exist for bringing electronic records to the students for learning in laboratories and classrooms. Although students in some schools gain experience charting in electronic charts and records in clinical settings, some schools now provide this type of learning experience in their classroom and clinical laboratory settings. These academic EHR systems can be used to create a wide range of fictitious patients, with many different medical issues, nursing needs, and personal/healthcare backgrounds. These records alone can be used to create a very complex patient for a case study or an entire unit of patients on which students can practice prioritizing critical thinking skills. In either case, these case records provide the context in which students see their "patients" and provide additional detail and history that can be used to develop students' critical thinking skills. Electronic records incorporating the patient health and medical history provide an added dimension to the snapshot of a patient that students gain during a simulated scenario. In an early example, the Simulated E-hEalth Delivery System (SEEDS) project (www.kumc.edu/health-informatics/seeds-in-use.html) was used in helping students gain this context. SEEDS used created patient cases in the clinical laboratory, showing students how to collect data, fill out standardized forms in created electronic charts, and then generate questions to identify potential patient problems. Projects such as SEEDS allow faculty to demonstrate first collection of data on individual patients and then data aggregation for the larger population. The Neehr Perfect Educational Electronic Health Record (neehrperfect.com) is another example of an academic EHRS valuable for student learning.

Further Resources to Support Informatics Teaching and Learning

Various tools exist to help educators incorporate informatics into their teaching. Respected projects such as the Quality and Safety Education for Nurses (QSEN) Institute, funded by The Robert Wood Johnson Foundation, provide specific student assignments relevant to informatics. Sample assignments include performing student self-assessments on informatics competencies (using rubrics); describing how nurses use informatics technology in their workplace, and addressing concepts such as administration, communication, data access, documentation, patient monitoring, quality improvement, and research.

Broad strategies, such as expanding connections with clinical practice partners to include informatics speakers and opportunities for demonstrating system capabilities, are recommended (NLN, 2015). The AACN (2008) recommends integrative student learning experiences with a range of technologies to support patient care, as well as student participation in quality assurance projects as a component of informatics.

Examples of Common Information Management Systems

Examples of standardized tools also are readily accessible on the Internet. The Long Term Care MDS is one example of an information management system with easy online access to data sets and information (see Exhibit 13.4). Faculty and students also have ready access to learn about other data sets. For beginning students, the introduction could include well-recognized data sets. Examples of electronic data resources with web resources and populations applications that might be used in classes include the following:

- The National Hospital Quality Measures (core measures) is used by The Joint Commission to monitor hospital quality.
- The NDNQI, maintained by the ANA, is used as a repository for nursing-sensitive indicators and outcomes (multiple hospitals submit data).
- The Functional Independence Measure (FIM) is the data set used to document disability and progress in rehabilitation settings.
- The Outcome and Assessment Information Set (OASIS) is the data set used in home healthcare to assess and monitor home care clients.
- The Long Term Care MDS provides a comprehensive electronic record for use in long-term care facilities.

EXHIBIT 13.4

LONG TERM CARE MINIMUM DATA SET EXEMPLAR

MDS, used in long-term care nursing facilities, can serve as an example to help students understand the potential of electronic records in healthcare. Students can easily gain examples of the assessment tool and its uses from reputable, government-supported websites.

The MDS has a long-standing history as an information system and ELR in long-term care. The MDS standardized assessment tool is used to collect data on all nursing home residents, on admission and at specified intervals, as part of an electronic record. The recorded data then provide information used to monitor quality care indicators such as weight loss or depression for individual facility residents. For example, data from a facility resident who has been losing weight over a 3-month period causes a flag on the electronic record, indicating that further attention to this problem is needed.

The information collected on individuals is then also combined to provide descriptive statistics on selected quality indicators for residents in the entire nursing home, state, or other geographic region. For example, a summary of the percentage of residents losing weight in one particular facility can be compared with percentages of residents losing weight in other facilities. Extensive data about specific nursing home resident variables can be gained when the right questions are asked of the MDS database. Reviewing the multiple uses for this tool with students can provide opportunity to begin discussions on electronic data management systems in general. Summary points include:

- At the resident level, the MDS includes basic resident assessment data completed on electronic records. These are called the *RAPs*. These RAPs then serve to organize data for generation of a standardized care plan for specific residents.
- Nursing homes also transmit MDS data electronically to a state-based MDS repository. Information is then captured at the CMS national database. This information feeds into quality indicators and reimbursement guides at state and federal levels.
- These grouped resident data then also feed into broad population information, allowing a type of benchmarking for long-term care facilities. Grouped resident assessment data on specific nursing home quality measures are posted at Nursing Home Compare (www.medicare.gov/nhcompare). Each facility's data can then be compared with other facilities' data (making it possible to provide information about facilities, such as percentage of residents with weight loss or depression, to families).

CMS, Centers for Medicare & Medicaid Services; EHR, electronic health record; MDS, Minimum Data Set; RAPs, Resident Assessment Protocols.

Any of these programs can be searched on the Internet for summaries of their tools, processes, and outcomes. Being aware of current approaches and where to learn more about them on the Internet can be a good starting point for students.

SUMMARY

Clinical data management tools, such as EHRs, enhance individual care within healthcare systems and focus population care. Our goal is to gain tools/ideas for using technology with our students to promote learning and ultimately safe, quality patient care. Students. as well as practicing professionals, will continue to need more exposure and training related to information management systems at all levels of their education. In summary, we can help students learn in the following ways:

- Considering individual electronic data that students collect on their patients, including how collected data (individual bits) can be combined to create a holistic picture of patient needs
- Learning about how data can be grouped to provide knowledge of characteristics, activities, and outcomes of large populations
- Learning about evidence-based standardized plans that are patient relevant and learning about outcome-based practice via automated clinical pathways to study care processes and outcomes
- Focusing on accurate data recording because this affects not only the patient health record, but also the administrative record relevant to issues such as diagnosis and billing codes
- Focusing on benefits of EHRs with standardized data that can be tracked over time and shared with multiple providers
- Using data at advanced student levels for answering evaluative and research questions

Although the tools we use will change, broad teaching learning principles assist students in gaining comfort with basic concepts and changing technologies. Health professions educators have the responsibility to prepare students of the future with a variety of tools that make them effective practitioners and team members. Changing technologies will be their tools as they work with patients for safe, effective quality care.

ENDING REFLECTIONS FOR YOUR LEARNING NOTEBOOK

1. What is the most important content that you learned in this chapter?
2. What are your plans for using the information provided in this chapter in your future teaching endeavors?
3. What are your further learning goals?

GUIDELINES FOR TEACHING AND LEARNING WITH TECHNOLOGIES

Quick Teaching Tips

1. Think about the varied ways electronic data are used in a familiar clinical agency and use these exemplars with students.
2. Help students learn about population health using online resources such as Healthy People 2020 in creating assignments.
3. Talk with clinical partners about their quality-improvement projects to help students gain exemplars of data management for improved patient care.

Questions for Further Reflection

NURSING INFORMATICS

1. How would you describe the term *nursing informatics* to a new faculty member or to a student?
2. What can help facilitate the incorporation of NI knowledge and skills into your nursing education curriculum?
3. What are the challenges of incorporating NI knowledge and skills into your nursing education curriculum?

ELECTRONIC HEALTH RECORDS

1. What are the best strategies for helping students gain experiences on EHRs? Academic settings? Clinical settings? Multiple clinic settings? Identify the pros and cons to each.
2. What are best practices in using information systems to assist students in promoting safe, quality patient care?

Learning Activity: Make a List

The purpose of this assignment is to help you as faculty think about the many ways you already use information management in your work with students. Make a list of the ways that you use (or will use) information management in working with students in your academic and clinical settings. What ways do technologies help you related to your work with students or staff? What ways do these relate to your work in educational administration, communication, documentation, and monitoring? Are there ways you can share examples with students?

Learning Activity: Create an Assignment

For your current or future students, generate an assignment that involves students considering a unique population with online data; for example, this could include describing the most prevalent health conditions in an area and then comparing them with state and national data. The purpose of this activity is to recall what you have learned in previous chapters and create an assignment to help students gain experience in accessing and using readily available data to describe select populations.

Online Resources for Further Learning

This resource review can help you gain ideas and resources for ongoing and future work. The following have particular reference in guiding clinical students:

- Technology Informatics Guiding Educational Reform (TIGER) Initiative (Health Information Technology). The TIGER group, a part of the HIMSS organization, have participated in developing targets for knowledge, skill, and attitude development during prelicensure education. www.himss.org/professionaldevelopment/tiger-initiative

- QSEN Institute This website provides extensive resources and sample assignments organized around safety, quality, and the additional recommended competencies of the IOM's (2003) health professions report, including informatics. www.qsen.org

REFERENCES

American Association of Colleges of Nursing. (2008). The essentials of baccalaureate education for professional nursing practice. Retrieved from http://www.aacnnursing.org/Portals/42/Publications/BaccEssentials08.pdf

Clancy, T. R. (2015). Integrating AACN Essentials for information management and patient care technologies across the continuum: Presentation, national nursing informatics deep dive program. Retrieved from https://www.nursing.umn.edu/sites/nursing.umn.edu/files/integrative-aacn-essentials-for-information-management.pdf

Coiera, E. (2015). Guide to health informatics (3rd ed.). Great Britain, UK: Hodder Arnold Publication.

Healthcare Information and Management Systems Society. (n.d.). The electronic health record. Retrieved from http://www.himss.org/ASP/index.asp

Hebda, T., & Czar, P. (2014). Handbook of informatics for nurses and health care professionals (2nd ed.). Saddle River, NJ: Prentice Hall.

Institute of Medicine. (2001). Crossing the quality chasm. A new health system for the 21st century. Washington, DC: National Academies Press.

Institute of Medicine. (2003). Health professions education: A bridge to quality. Washington, DC: National Academies Press.

McGonigle, D., & Mastrian, K. (2017). Informatics for health professionals. Boston, MA: Jones & Bartlett.

National League for Nursing Board of Governors. (2015). A vision for the changing faculty role: Preparing students for the technological world of health care. Retrieved from https://www.nln.org/docs/default-source/about/nln-vision-series-(position-statements)/a-vision-for-the-changing-faculty-role-preparing-students-for-the-technological-world-of-health-care.pdf?sfvrsn=0

The Joint Commission. (2017). Performance measurement initiatives. Retrieved from https://www.jointcommission.org/performance_measurement.aspx

U.S. Department of Health and Human Services. (2003). Summary of the HIPAA privacy rule. Retrieved from http://www.hhs.gov/ocr/privacy/hipaa/understanding/summary/index.html

Winstanley, H. D. (2017). A qualitative descriptive study exploring associate degree nursing faculty's experiences teaching electronic health record systems use (Doctoral dissertation). University of Kansas Medical Center, Kansas City, KS.

CHAPTER 14

Technology and Clinical Teaching and Learning: Creating a Culture of Safety

CHAPTER GOAL

Guide students in using technologies to provide safe, quality care in clinical settings.

BEGINNING REFLECTION

What experiences (as an educator or student) have you had in using clinical technologies in the following ways? What are your best or most challenging experiences?

1. Considering diverse technologies and student learning needs in the clinical setting?
2. Identifying best practices for teaching students to use technology in the clinical setting?
3. Creating assignments that address student learning needs for safe, quality clinical care?

Overheard: *What If our students make a medication mistake? How should we handle that?*

Clinical experiences are central in creating nursing providers. Healthcare education has always been distinguished in preparing students to care for patients in actual clinical settings. This unique clinical practice brings many opportunities and challenges in using technology when working with students. A number of Institute of Medicine (IOM) safety reports have made clear that faculty need to play a major role in developing students who provide safe care to patients. Technology has been identified as a central tool for promoting safe, quality patient care and supporting a clinical culture of safety (IOM Committee on the Health Professions Education, 2003). More opportunities exist for developing optimal pedagogy and technology combinations for clinical laboratories and actual clinical care settings. In the past, students went to the classroom and clinical practicum with limited technology resources for learning. Now students have access to numerous electronic books and Internet resources in preparing for clinical patient care. In the past, faculty often prepared students for their clinical experiences with some role play–type activity in the clinical laboratory rather than with the high-fidelity patient simulator or virtual gaming that now provides opportunities for learning safe clinical practice. We now have opportunities to be creative with a variety of technology resources in learning what works best to develop safe practitioners.

Knowledge gained in the classroom needs to be applied in clinical settings while keeping patients safe and cared for effectively. This chapter helps us think about how best to use technology in organizing teaching for our clinically focused outcomes. As changes occur in both clinical laboratories and the hospital setting, how can technology assist faculty in developing safe healthcare professionals? This chapter discusses pedagogies for supporting technology as a tool in the changing clinical laboratories and in the clinical units and agencies. It also discusses technology as a tool for caring for patients at the point of care.

PEDAGOGY AND THE CHANGING CLINICAL LEARNING LABORATORY

The clinical laboratory provides a structured teaching environment where students can learn safe application of skills, as well as critical thinking. It provides a setting for helping students learn about and promote safety awareness. Practicing this culture of safety begins in the clinical laboratory, which prepares students for their current and future roles in promoting safe, quality care. In addition, it includes faculty modeling professional behaviors for students, as well as providing diverse simulation opportunities and addressing potential safety issues in both acute and home care settings.

The clinical learning laboratory, a resource for multiple health providers, offers a variety of teaching and learning opportunities. Teaching devices range from simple mannequins to electronic arms for practicing intravenous injection to authentically simulated patients. Practice laboratories provide opportunities for students to gain comfort with a variety of challenging skills such as intravenous starts, nasogastric tube insertion, intubation, and blood administration. The learning laboratory takes on increasing importance with access to high-fidelity patient simulations that provide students with real-time practice in intense or high-risk situations that would be limited in the real-world clinical setting.

Learning laboratories are unique settings with tools and resources that vary by school from low- to high-technology sites. Some laboratories mimic hospital settings in appearance, and others include clinic rooms and home-based simulations. In many, high-fidelity patient simulators have become important tools and have led to whole families of simulators. Galloway (2009) provides an extensive discussion of the types of simulator technologies found to provide students with safe practice and learning opportunities.

The pedagogy of clinical teaching incorporates applied learning. Consistent with classroom teaching, faculty assess learners' needs and match assignments to class objectives, focusing on the interactive learning opportunities available in the laboratory setting. It involves identifying students' strengths and weaknesses, as well as providing assignments that promote practice and build student confidence and safety. Clinical learning laboratories also provide opportunities for increased focus on self-directed learning and documentation of student competencies.

How do faculty best use technology to organize effective clinical preparation experiences that prepare students for safe clinical practice? Questions to consider for the clinical laboratory include the following:

- What are the benefits of laboratory practice? How much practice and "actual" clinical experience are needed?
- What do we mean by "student practice" and how will it be structured?
- How many ways are there to help students learn with technology in the learning laboratory? How real and safe can faculty make these experiences?
- What are the requirements for student preparation for the learning laboratory? How prepared should faculty expect students to be before walking in the door?

The clinical learning laboratory can provide a functional, supportive environment for learning. For the laboratory to be effective and efficient, attention must be paid to the design of the setting of learning activities and to the support staff in the laboratory (from faculty to teaching assistants). All of these individuals must use good principles of teaching and learning as they work with students on clinical laboratory assignments. Sample approaches for promoting success in the clinical laboratory, no matter what technology is used, include orienting students to their roles, clearly identifying laboratory purposes, and determining rubrics to guide learning.

Orienting Students to Clinical Laboratory Learning Assignments

Faculty can help students understand the expectations for each clinical laboratory assignment by guiding students in preparation it (e.g., clarity on preparation expectations, including reading assignments and practice activities prior to the laboratory. In the past, faculty used class time to watch videos and practice in the laboratory. Now if we choose, we can have students "prewatch" an orientation online. Preparing for the clinical laboratory becomes a new experience with the variety of teaching and learning aids available online. Although benefits exist to these online resources, potential challenges also exist if students seek their own Internet resources that may not have been critiqued or peer reviewed. Appropriate guidelines for such reviews then become a part of the clinical learning orientation.

Ideally, students come to the laboratory ready to apply what they have read ahead of time and have more time to apply knowledge and work on skills. If there is student "down" time in the laboratory, having learning activities, such as mobile-device assignments, while students are waiting to be checked off on a skill promotes use of learning time.

Identifying Laboratory Purposes and Effective Assignment Design

In terms of overall planning, setting specific objectives for learning laboratory sessions is central. Effective assignments are guided by session objectives. With use of the Integrated Learning Triangle for Teaching With Technologies (Exhibit 1.3), the concepts of assessment, appropriate learning activities, and evaluation come together. Determining whether the learning laboratory assignment is for practice and whether it will include a summative grade is considered in the planning phase. Walvoord and Anderson (2009) note the importance of this determination and students' awareness prior to evaluation. As you orient yourself and others to the technologies of the learning laboratory, consider the following:

- How is technology best used to help with laboratory check-offs and monitoring of student progression?
- Is the laboratory time scheduled with faculty available to provide instruction as students practice?
- Is the laboratory time a student solo effort or do students assist one another with assigned roles?
- Are procedure check-offs required? Are students required to share the theory/rationale that supports the behaviors they demonstrate?
- Are check-offs completed by faculty or a teaching assistant? Are check-offs completed by peers acceptable? Can self-assessment and peer review be part of check-offs?
- Are laboratory check-offs just skills checklists or do they include making a "chart note" related to the case study/clinical skill? There are advantages to having students access and learn recording procedures with electronic health records to help prepare them for clinical patient care.

Guiding Clinical Laboratories With Rubrics and Checklists

Providing skills checklists for students provides direction in their skill learning and practice. Rubrics or checklists are beneficial in facilitating both the laboratory experience and the clinical grading for faculty and students. They promote clear communication as to expectations of best practice in completing skills. Rubrics help in clearly outlining expectation for students. This is especially important in seeking to promote a culture of safety in clinical practice. Faculty discussion about these tools and how they are to be used can promote best practices. There can be differences in how these tools are interpreted, so when they are used for student evaluation by multiple faculty, aiming for inter-rater reliability is important for promoting fairness in evaluation. Moreover, students can use these tools for self-assessments and peer assessments to promote learning.

Within learning management systems, these checklists can be distributed to students, as well as checked off and tracked or monitored for competencies. As noted, important faculty decisions include the type of rubrics and checklists to be used and how they are to be used.

Using Technology to Plan Clinical Experiences

The clinical setting is complex with busy staff, anxious students, and often, complicated patient care. For clinical staff, there may be challenges working with students related to multiple schools, varied levels of students, varied assignments, and a variety of staff and health professionals. Helping staff in the clinical settings better understand faculty plans and student needs provides a good start to the clinical experience. Thinking about clinical education as a link between education and practice can promote ease of planning. Technology can be used for sharing clinical resources. Benefits exist for a central online resource for housing orientation materials that staff and students can access. Websites can be used to facilitate the clinical experiences in the following ways:

- *Initial organizing*. Many schools and hospitals have formed partnerships, using the Internet as a tool for scheduling students, to promote optimal student numbers for patient care.
- *Document repository*. Websites provide spots for housing the clinical learning documents, evaluation guidelines, and student rosters with needed information.
- *Ongoing communication*. Providing online access to clinical tools for staff and preceptors can not only promote ease in accessing student resources, but also enhance communication with clinicians.

Sharing needed clinical tools and accessing preceptors using technology promotes team communication. An example of an online studio developed for doctorate of nursing practice (DNP) preceptors is described in Exhibit 14.1.

EXHIBIT 14.1

CASE EXAMPLE: ONLINE DNP PRECEPTOR STUDIO

Compiled by: Diane Ebbert, PhD, APRN
Moya Peterson, PhD, APRN, FNP-BC

The importance of well-prepared preceptors in socializing advanced practice nursing students is clear. Although DNP programs are being developed by various schools and organizations, preceptor training of DNPs has not been well addressed. This case example

(continued)

describes the Online DNP Preceptor Studio, part of a DNP postmaster's program at the University of Kansas. A system's framework of structure, process, and outcomes organized the development of this studio. The Preceptor Studio, a web-based resource, is designed to assist advance practice preceptors gain or update teaching skills.

The structure of the resource (including the studio format and available preceptor resources), the studio development process (including focus group data from practitioners), and outcomes (evaluative data, including preceptor use of resources, self-assessment scores, and studio/resource satisfaction) are shared online. Adult education principles, evidence-based practices from multiple disciplines, and National Organization of Nurse Practitioner Faculties inform the precepting resources. Tools such as best-practice tools for personal mobile devices, web-based resources for fingertip knowledge, and resources for coaching and mentoring are part of this resource. The online studio is unique in preparing the much-needed clinicians/preceptors for applying evidence-based practice at the bedside and gaining coping skills in new preceptor roles. This just-in-time learning resource provides tools and ideas useful in other programs as well.

DNP, Doctorate of nursing practice.

FACULTY ORIENTATION TO CLINICAL UNITS AND TECHNOLOGY

As faculty preparing to take students to clinical units, we want to be as familiar as possible with these settings. Gaining familiarity includes exploring the clinical unit and determining the learning team participants (clinical facility staff, instructors, students, patients, and college partners). Reviewing clinical unit Internet resources and having needed names and contact information available electronically promote ease of communication. Technologies can provide faculty support in gaining familiarity with clinical units and organizing the first days of class and clinical experiences, as well as providing opportunities to engage staff as partners in educating our clinical students. Sample technology considerations for clinical faculty include the following:

- What broad technology resources and tools will be used by students? For example, what technologies will be used for medication administration and access of the medication system?
- What electronic health records are used and what system is used for students to access needed records?

STUDENT ORIENTATIONS

Beginning a clinical experience involves setting a positive climate, both physically and emotionally, for student learning. Helping students move from clinical laboratory technologies to hands-on caring is a key faculty endeavor. The goal is to help students gain comfort, increase skills, and be safe in the clinical setting. Orienting students to their roles and the setting is important in helping them gain comfort, thus minimizing their anxiety as they begin their clinical learning. In a given clinical setting, technology can help organize an effective orientation organized around the important concepts of place, people, and process.

Instructors help students understand each of the following concepts: the physical structure and resources of an emergency room, the process and protocols for providing care, and the expected patient outcomes and the ways that the outcomes are documented.

- **The Place**. Orientation to place involves gaining familiarity with and comfort in the physical environment, including the layout and the resources. Can electronic documents be distributed to students that will promote this? Can videos of units be shown to provide an introductory orientation? Are in-house electronic resources available to provide information about laboratory, diagnostic, and pharmacy resources?
- **The Process**. Orientation to the process involves identifying how things are done on the unit and how students can participate. Are selected staff willing to provide a brief welcome video to students, sharing their philosophy of the clinical unit?
- **The People**. Orientation to people means being introduced to key staff with whom students will be working. Are there electronic repositories with staff introductions or professional social networks that students can use to gain introductions?

The clinical syllabus serves as an orientation tool and can be outlined and shared electronically with students and staff. Additional ideas for orienting students include electronic introductory letters (to both students and staff), tours (video or face to face), and scavenger hunts (electronic or face to face).

FACILITATING AND SUPERVISING WORK WITH STUDENTS

The clinical setting brings unique challenges because students bring their own anxieties and stresses to busy, complex clinical units with diverse patient needs. As students move into the actual clinical setting, our goal is to integrate technology and other resources for promoting student and patient clinical safety, building on what students learned in the clinical laboratory. How do faculty keep up with their many students and their patients' medications, treatments, diagnostic tests, and clinical procedures? Beginning approaches include using technology, such as in the following ways, to plan clinical experiences:

- Online resources or electronic distribution of resource materials
- Web-based tools to access students' postclinical write-ups or reflective journals
- Online discussions for postclinical sharing and debriefing
- Electronic management systems, including tracking systems, such as Typhon, that track the types of patient care experiences that students have had and generate reports that summarize cumulative clinical experiences

What is the best way to keep track of students who are correlating content for critical thinking and safe care of patients? Coaching and supervising using technology includes maintaining good communication with students.

This process often involves issues with multiple units and communications with both students and resource clinicians. Technology provides help such as increased access to preceptors, mobile devices for clinical logs, and technology through which students can check in and follow up with faculty.

Mobile computing devices are efficient tools for faculty organization. This technology, a type of automated notebook or clipboard, serves as an organizing tool for faculty to support supervision responsibilities. Examples of ways that mobile computing devices such as tablets can help faculty organize include the following:

- Electronic assignment grids for organizing clinical days with students
- Reminder systems for tracking students and procedures
- Tools for quick clinical notes such as student anecdotal records

Mobile devices also serve as information resources that help guide students in evidence-based practice, providing access to portable texts and online resources to an evidence base for confirming plans and approaches. As students learn new medications, these tools help them confirm dosages, alerting them to potential problems or side effects. This clinical technology has the benefits of promoting patient safety and organizing large amounts of information. New uses of video with these pockettype devices are also being developed. Exhibit 14.2 provides a case example using point-of-care instant teacher (POCIT) videos. In addition, the Health Insurance Portability and Accountability Act (HIPAA) privacy issues in clinical settings and the need for password protection are noted.

EXHIBIT 14.2

CASE EXAMPLE: POCIT VIDEOS: POINT-OF-CARE INSTANT TEACHER

Compiled by: Mary N. Meyer, PhD, APRN and Sharon Kumm, MN, RN, CNE

In a rapidly changing clinical environment, students are faced with multiple ways of performing basic procedures. Although procedures change in response to new research findings, change at the bedside may lag behind the evidence. To complicate matters, there is frequently more than one *correct* way to perform basic nursing procedures. Even when students accept more than one "right way" as acceptable, they are frustrated when teaching is inconsistent.

Requiring mobile devices for our undergraduate nursing students for the past several years, we wanted to expand their learning opportunities beyond the traditional textbooks. A faculty member proposed the idea of producing digital videos of techniques that could be accessed on mobile devices by students to review in clinical settings. In addition to providing instant access to best practice, the videos might encourage the student to share the best practice with staff nurses or use the videos as a patient teaching aid. After a faculty and student survey as to the most needed videos was conducted, five videos varying from tracheostomy care to insertion of

(continued)

intravenous catheters were developed. The process for video development included the use of current evidence from the literature for script development. Graduate teaching assistants volunteered to be the actors, and the institution's instructional support department assisted with filming, voice-over, and editing of the digital product. Videos were stored on the online learning management system, allowing students to access and download them from several courses. Faculty encouraged students to access the videos.

After project implementation of the first semester, approval was gained from the institution's institutional review board for a student and faculty survey on project satisfaction. Excep for students' wanting more orientation for accessing the videos, other comments indicated favorable satisfaction with the videos. This project was developed with support from the NLN HITS program.

HITS, Health Information Technology Scholars; NLN, National League for Nursing.

TECHNOLOGY AND DOCUMENTING FOR LEARNING

Clinical care and documentation are intertwined. Critical thinking is enhanced as students determine what information to pass on to their patient team. Technologies can help in orienting students to clinical preparation and documentation expectations. The following questions can guide thinking about particular pedagogies:

- What type of preparation sheets, care plans, or concept maps will students be completing on assigned patients? What questions should they be prepared to answer for evidence-based care? What technologies can support their work in these areas?
- How are students best prepared to communicate with the team? What ways are students best challenged to gain skill with the situation-background-assessment-recommendation (SBAR) technique? How does this help prepare for electronic documentation?
- What documentation systems will students be using in working with their patients? What guidelines do students need? Electronic health records, also discussed in Chapter 13, are a central part of learning.
- Electronic health record systems play a central role for students in learning documentation. As discussed further in Chapter 13, access to these EHR systems for patient care documentation presents challenges in some cases but is a needed skill (and legal requirement) for all practicing nurses.

CONFERENCING AND DEBRIEFING

The purpose of the postclinical conference is to debrief and assist students in reflecting on and learning from their experiences. The reflection on practice or reflective practice that a postclinical debriefing allows fits well with technologies. Literature on simulations has highlighted the importance of these postclinical debriefings (National League for Nursing [NLN], 2015).

Arranging mutual times and locations for postclinical conferences can be challenging. Using electronic methods can ease this challenge, with online resources providing an alternate approach to traditional face-to-face clinical conferencing. Technology can help here in the following ways:

- Debriefing online can include student journals or clinical day summaries completed electronically and shared with faculty via electronic methods such as email or learning management systems.
- Clinical narratives based on Benner's model (Erickson, Ditomassi, Sabia, & Smith, 2015) shared in electronic portfolio format provide students with an opportunity to name what they are doing. Using precourse and then postcourse narratives encourages students to note their advancing skills (seeking higher-order practice across the semester).
- Preconferences can also use technology to help assess learner readiness and help learners prioritize their learning needs/goals. Faculty might conduct preconferences online when necessary.

USING TECHNOLOGIES IN CLINICAL EVALUATION

Clinical evaluation is enhanced by technology. Once faculty have organized a good clinical experience for students, technology can help provide clinical feedback on written work, patient care observations, or even distant site clinical experiences. Broad evaluation concepts build on the American Association for Higher Education assessment guidelines (Hutchings, Ewell, & Banta, 2012) and are further discussed in Chapter 9. These guidelines include specific approaches and rationale for student evaluation tools such as evaluative data that combine reflections, written work/examinations, and clinical observations and involve multiple reviewers when possible. Technology can help with the following:

- Triangulating evaluation methods and evaluators with increased use of clinical learning laboratories in competency checks.
- Tracking of minimum safety competencies; electronic systems can be used in in the learning laboratory check-offs.
- Making best uses of clinical rubrics for evaluation of student written work.
- Amassing multiple sources of data for evaluation: student report, patient report, staff report, observation, and record review.
- Helping students develop skills in self-assessment and peer review (e.g., students may do self-assessments and peer check-offs against a rubric as practice for a final). Peer feedback and teamwork are consistent with recommendations from the Quality and Safety Education for Nurses (QSEN) Institute for helping students gain additional team-focused learning (QSEN, 2017).
- Completing summative evaluations with input from the learner (e.g., inviting the learner's self-assessment in electronic format, comparing this with faculty summation, and using any differences as points for further discussion).

- Sharing electronic preceptor evaluation and site evaluation tools for students to complete. Clinical tracking systems, as noted earlier, exist in which students' clinical experiences, the number of hours spent, the preceptors used, the facilities visited, and the objectives met can all be logged and documented. These systems can track students across their entire academic programs, documenting the types of patients they see, the procedures they complete, and their progress from course to course. They simplify record keeping and save faculty time. Ease of use, cost, and faculty valuing of the system are factors in choosing the best tracking systems (Squires, 2009). As noted in Chapter 13, assignments can be developed for patient tracking systems and completed by students to further engage them in completing meaningful assignments and better understanding their patient populations.

Considering Technologies for Promoting Student and Staff Safety

A culture of safety, supported by numerous national safety and error reports, indicates a clear priority for all healthcare agencies. In preparing students for clinical activities, faculty want to stress the importance of a culture of safety. This involves addressing opportunities to enhance student safety in working with faculty and clinical partners as they care for patients. Sample approaches to consider in teaching and learning opportunities for students include:

- Safe environment. One strategy/approach is to help students advocate for a safe environment that minimizes falls and patient harm. Although many fall-prevention plans focus on the patient's physical status, including diagnoses and medication, many external environmental factors such as room design and special equipment can also contribute. Although technologies have obvious value in patient rooms, sometimes basic safety concerns, such as excess clutter and electrical cords, are missed. One strategy includes having students do initial room scans for each patient, using a basic checklist that includes items such as environmental fall hazards that can be easily fixed.
- Safe lifting. Large percentages of nursing staff suffer musculoskeletal injuries related to unsafe lifting practices, sometimes even leaving the profession due to back pain. In addition to nurse injury, patients can also fall and/or or be injured by poor transfer techniques. Body mechanics alone are no longer considered safe lifting methods, so safe lifting devices, a type of basic technology, are available for helping students learn. A comprehensive program for safe lifting involves establishment of policies, equipment and training guidelines, and program evaluation (American Nurses Association, 2013).
- Teamwork for safety. A climate of respect sets the stage for safe quality care for all. The goal for creating a learning climate of respect, is for all team members to work together in being accountable to a system that decreases adverse care events and promotes quality care. Interprofessional

education (IPE) competencies, based on best evidence, have been developed to help move this effort forward (Interprofessional Education Collaborative, 2016). Collaboration and communication among multiple disciplines are important competencies in these standards. When working as part of a team, all members should positively role model professional behaviors. This includes communicating with respectful language, as well as communicating with clear, confident approaches using common language that all would understand.

Creating a culture of safety also includes addressing error (actual or potential) from a broad system's perspective (Lachman, 2015). In the past, students were typically "in trouble" for a safety incident (and so might fail to report them). A culture of safety supports reporting and learning from incidents or near misses. For example, if a student incident such as a medication error occurred (no trauma to the patient, but a concern), should student blame and repercussions follow? What ways could this be approached to promote improvements for the future, consistent with a culture of safety? Sample points to consider include:

- Do students know the safety basics and what to do if an event occurs? What are the unit's structure and process for safe medication administration? What student and staff communication issues need to be addressed to prevent future problems?
- If an error occurs, do students know the reporting procedure (including appropriate channels starting with faculty?) Their role in taking responsibility?
- How is the situation best debriefed with students and staff (the what, so what, and now what?), clarifying, for example, what led to the problem. What communication and systems issues contributed (were the right people, the right resources, and the right environmental factors in place)? What changes in the system need to be made to prevent this problem another time?

TECHNOLOGIES FOR ASSISTING PATIENTS AT POINT OF CARE

Technologies are pervasive in clinical care. Devices are as basic as electronic thermometers and blood pressure devices purchased at local drug stores. They include accessing evidence-based resources and clinical decision systems at the point of care. Clinical technology tools can include telephones for verbal monitoring of patient progress and digital cameras to monitor wound progression. Guiding and evaluating students in technology-rich clinical settings are central faculty roles.

At the point of care, there are all kinds of technologies for students to gain comfort with. Students are introduced to devices that translate patients' basic physiological functions to screens and printouts for monitoring patient care.

From monitors to tubes and central lines, the opportunities for learning with technology are extensive. The American Association of Colleges of Nursing (AACN) *Essentials* specifically address the need for student learning about applications of clinical care technology (AACN, 2008).

Critical care and surgical care settings provide good examples of extensive technologies for monitoring patients and supporting their care needs. Even general hospital units often resemble the critical care units of years past. Technologies are also key features in home care. Technologies that support patient care include patient monitoring equipment, drug and intravenous system alerts, and patient identification systems such as bar coding. They are therefore considered essential in nursing education (AACN, 2008). Students must gain comfort with numerous technologies at the point of care.

All tools, including technologies such as cardiac monitors and respirators that have been a part of clinical experiences for many years, are new to students at some point. In getting our students ready for the work world, we can use basic approaches to teaching these technologies that can begin in the clinical laboratory. For all types of technology, students need to know the basic purposes, ways to monitor for correct function, and troubleshooting of problems. Students gain comfort with the technology "parts," as well as the evidence-based protocols that guide their use.

Safe and prudent use of technology includes what Benner et al. (2011) described as practical technology assessments. In their discussion of technology in the critical care setting, the authors note that practical technology assessments include determining its usefulness for a particular patient, appropriate safety factors, and protocols for accurate management and interpreting equipment performance readings correctly. The authors described both caring and ethical considerations, in technology as well as its safe use. In addition to learning how a particular technology works and how to interpret the data provided, students need to consider how to blend caring and direct hands-on care ("high touch") with technologies. Students are reminded how important it is to care for the patient and not focus just on the technologies. Strategies as basic as the positioning of computer screens to promote optimal contact with patients can make a difference.

Although not all new nurses will specialize in clinical areas where patient care technology is extensive, opportunities exist for all students to learn the basics of safe, reasonable care according to standards. Concerns have emerged about the frequency of technology work-arounds, a term used when bypassing technology-based patient protocols (e.g., with medication administration). Work-arounds are fraught with competing expectations for nurses and the students who are watching them. Faculty need to help students see that "quick fixes" that bypass the technology protocol can put patients at safety risk and violate a nurse's professional obligation to follow the rules (Berlinger, 2017).

Faculty can create introductory assignments that allow students to gain comfort with a range of technologies. For example, faculty could start a class by asking students to brainstorm how many ways they use technologies in patient care. This discussion can then be extended to include questions that help students address the benefits and challenges of selected technologies. Exhibit 14.3

EXHIBIT 14.3

SAMPLE ASSIGNMENTS FOR ENHANCING STUDENT TECHNOLOGY AWARENESS IN THE CLINICAL SETTING

- Ask students to brainstorm types of technologies patients/families can purchase at the local drugstore, such as basic electronic thermometers and blood pressure devices.
- Ask students to think of times they have used technologies as monitoring devices, such as pulse oximetry or ECG rhythm strips.
- Ask students to review online product resources, both written and video, to prepare for their clinical experiences.
- Have students make a survey of the tools/technologies they will be using in a clinical rotation, such as central line transducers, ventilators, fetal monitoring equipment, or remote telemetry. Include Internet resources that provide product reviews or divide students into groups and ask them to share a product summary from the Internet.
- Use the Internet for clinical preparation. Students learn new clinical technologies by reviewing online product resources, both written and video. Herrman (2015) describes the "equipment conference" in which students focus on learning the mechanics and the clinician role in using technologies that are new to them.
- Assign students to work with expert staff and observe these tools being used efficiently and appropriately.
- Have students discuss issues regarding electronic medication management, including topics such as order entry, management, and pharmacy tracking.
- Bring videos of the clinical setting to classrooms for large group orientations, especially when orienting students to settings such as the emergency room or operating room that may be less available for in-person orientations.

provides additional examples related to technologies awareness in the clinical setting and potential needs for orientation and safety discussions.

Although a goal for students is competent practice, often a reasonable starting point is in observing others at work on a select task or process. The reflective observer role, as supported in a descriptive study by Bonnel and Hober (2016), serves as one tool for enhancing learning by watching others. Although this study took place in the learning laboratory, opportunities exist to extend reflective observer roles to select clinical setting (or even online videos of these settings). Reflective prompts, developed to direct students to select learning outcomes are a key feature of the observer assignments. These observer roles have opportunity for further development in peer-review and team-focused learning, important considerations for interprofessional teamwork. Implications for further implementation and evaluation related to the observer role include the following:

- Consider clinical and laboratory opportunities in which the observer role could serve as an important first step in learning (reflecting on a laboratory scenario of team roles in safety, collaboration, and communication as an example).
- Orient and facilitate all in using best reflection practices with observer assignments.

- Enhance tools for the observer, including reflective prompts to provide observer guidance on learning goals such as describing nursing or team roles and actions.
- Consider providing basic coaching on peer-review strategies and extending the observer role to a peer reviewer role in debriefings.

Exhibit 14.3 suggests sample assignments for enhancing technology awareness in the clinical setting.

TAKING CLINICAL LEARNING ONLINE

In some cases, clinical opportunities are lacking or do not easily meet all learning objectives. In this case, creative use of virtual cases is a possibility. Examples such as the Advancing Care Excellence for Seniors (ACES) program provide developed cases that can be adapted to meet student needs. Online virtual case coordination activities are additional assignment ideas (NLN, 2018). Chapter 16 also addresses approaches for a clinical practicum to accompany online courses.

Advancing clinical skills using online tools is another consideration in clinical learning. Students graduate from basic programs and need to continue lifelong learning, both to keep up with basic practice changes (continuing education requirements) and to extend their skills to more advanced specialty care. Megha Bonnel describes how she prepared her e-portfolio to help document her ongoing education and working toward a certification in her clinical specialty. She shares her experiences, combining her work with interprofessional colleague mentors and ongoing learning and development, that uses a technology focus and an e-portfolio to help document her ongoing learning (Exhibit 14.4)

EXHIBIT 14.4

LEARNING AN ADVANCED PRACTICE SPECIALTY

Megha Bonnel, APRN, MSN

1. ***What is your current position as an advanced practice nurse? How is technology involved?*** I work as an APRN in a urology specialty, working collaboratively with a physician. We see patients across diverse settings, including rehabilitation and acute care hospitals. We are in diverse settings, so we use online technologies and electronic records to review previous notes, imaging, and laboratory findings for patients. The challenges are that we must have images clouded to us, we do not have access to all records from all settings, and not all people are tech savvy.

   Recently our practice wanted to update our information and gain practices on PSA testing. I spent time reviewing various articles for new testing for prostate

(continued)

cancer. I summarized the articles and used them to help update our plans of care and protocols in the office. I was surprised how fast this diagnosing and treatment for prostate cancers seems to be constantly changing. It seems to relate to the rapid increase in genetics information. Also related to technology, right now, I am learning a new dictation system to increase the effectiveness of our documentation. I am helping troubleshoot and figure out if this is a technology that works for the team.

2. ***What ways did your education and educational technology help you prepare for this role?*** After completing my RN to BSN online, I completed my online graduate programs (nurse management and nurse practitioner). Even though the programs were online, they all used clinical practicums, and many of my courses used reflective assignments so that I could also relate new information to my work setting. I created an e-portfolio–type resource in a word-processing program and kept the reflective writing assignments about my practicum experiences. Even in early RN to BSN work, a diabetes educator helped me think about grouping my populations so that I had evidence practices for children, as well as adults and older adults. In my management program, my preceptor helped me gain best practices for an experienced clinical nurse specialist; it helped seeing how she used technologies in working with the physicians. Also, I recall reflections about working with an NP preceptor in long-term care and in ways to stay calm when dealing with complex situations (and nursing home technologies). In my graduate NP program, Typhon was a tool to help log or track patients I was seeing. It seemed challenging at the time to document all the individual patients seen, but then it was neat to use the reports function and be able to summarize the groups or populations of patients I was seeing, which was often surprising.

3. ***How do you stay current in your specialty? How is technology involved?*** Being part of the nurse urology organization been helpful. I get their electronic newsletters and journals. I belong to their association and attend their annual conference on a regular schedule and appreciate the electronic resources that they provide before and after these meetings. When I have time to work on my continuing education hours, I like to do webinars or podcasts because they are really convenient to help me stay current and gain hours. Also, my physician and other APRNs in our practice share articles and electronic updates that pertain to our practice. Electronic portfolios help me organize this. I also keep an electronic portfolio to document my education hours for continuing education and preparing for specialty certification.

4. ***Do you have any tips for others learning a practice specialty?*** My tip is to look up the information you do not understand and write it down to learn (I use an electronic notebook to keep track). Although most nursing programs start you out as a generalist, as mine did, it is really worth the effort to learn a specialty. I also think it is helpful to have a specialty certification examination to help you stay on track with your continuing education.

APRN, advanced practice registered nurse; PSA, prostate-specific antigen.

USING TECHNOLOGY IN GUIDING PATIENT EDUCATION

As further discussed in Chapter 15, students need to be well versed in technology that supports patient education. In a rapidly changing healthcare world, diverse patients cope with complex problems in less structured settings such as their homes. Technology allows more opportunities for gaining information to promote self-management. As patients assume more responsibility for their own care and well-being, one of the most important things nurses do to provide safety and quality care is patient education.

At this time of urgent need for patient education, technology offers many opportunities for supporting patients and families. It also offers many challenges as patients go to the Internet and find a variety of resources, some evidence based and many not. Students take on new roles in learning to guide their patients in appropriate uses of web resources for healthcare. Learning to critique web resources as students (as discussed in Chapter 5) now extends to helping patients learn to recognize quality resources when they search the Internet on their own.

In addition to freely accessible health-related Internet resources, a variety of clinical agencies now provide their own website directed at patient support. Thede and Sewell (2015) noted these websites often include a variety of resources such as message boards, chat rooms, email lists, or some combination of these. Sometimes, online support groups are also found within these venues, bringing their own unique issues, such as whether or not sites are moderated and who has access. Guiding students as they share evidence-based websites and help their patients learn basic website critique is a beginning step in improving patient knowledge.

SUMMARY

Clinical experiences serve as opportunities to integrate theory into practice. Clinical faculty have the opportunity to model best practices and build student confidence and self-esteem as members of the profession. From clinical learning with laboratory innovations and multiple types of simulations to clinical learning with varied technologies, the faculty role includes guiding students in the safe and effective use of many technologies. A focus includes monitoring both potential and actual safety hazards in the technology-rich clinical environment.

The patient care setting is where opportunities for theoretical and clinical learning come together. Pedagogies of adult education and the Integrated Learning Triangle for Teaching with Technologies (Exhibit 1.3) provide direction in both using technology and helping students learn. Teaching and learning with clinical technologies helps provide students with opportunities to integrate theory into practice and to enhance patient care.

ENDING REFLECTION FOR YOUR LEARNING NOTEBOOK

1. What is the most important content that you learned in this chapter?
2. What are your plans for using the information provided in this chapter in your future teaching endeavors?
3. What are your further learning goals?

GUIDELINES FOR TEACHING AND LEARNING WITH TECHNOLOGIES

Quick Teaching Tips

1. For students new to mobile device use in the clinical setting, develop quick pocket assignments that help them gain comfort in looking up medications, unique diagnoses, and other relevant clinical topics during any downtime in a clinical setting.
2. Use electronic concept mapping tools for students to map issues that relate to technology and patient safety.
3. Maximize student learning by reflective sharing of clinical experiences at postconference and through follow-up electronic journaling.

Questions for Further Reflection

1. What strategies can help faculty promote safe students and clinical practitioners? How much time do students need to spend in the clinical laboratory?
2. How do we best teach our students to gain "fingertip knowledge" with mobile devices? What are the benefits and the challenges of using the Internet in clinical education?
3. Should mobile devices be required in educational programs? What are the benefits and challenges of mobile devices in promoting student independence and patient safety?
4. How is your institution currently teaching students the importance of a clinical culture of safety? What additional strategies would you suggest to promote student clinical safety?
5. What ways might patient safety be compromised by disruptive staff behavior? What technology-related examples can you provide? What recommendations from the IPE competencies (IPEC, 2016) can help promote a safety culture?

Learning Activity: Preparing for Clinical

What if new clinical educators headed to their first day of clinical experience with no orientation regarding their role, no mentor, no grading rubric, no course objectives, and no student contact information? What if they did not know how to access electronic medical records or the electronic medication system and were not sure if the group had a conference room assigned to them? What problems would exist in this scenario? If you were preparing to work with students on a new clinical unit or helping orient new faculty, how would you use technologies to help address the following questions?

1. What should I include in the students' orientation to the clinical agency?
2. How do I orient myself to the clinical agency?

3. How do I initiate and maintain good relationships with staff at the clinical agency?

4. How do I (and students) access clinical technologies such as electronic health records and medications (including needed student codes)?

Learning Activity: Creating an Assignment

As you think about sharing, with your students, resources regarding creating a culture of safety, review selected resources such as those provided by the Agency for Healthcare Research and Quality (AHRQ) modules, *Understand the Science of Safety*. As you review selected modules, your purpose is to help determine which resources can best be used in your teaching and creation of student assignments (www.ahrq.gov/professionals/education/curriculum-tools/cusptoolkit/modules/understand/index.html).

Online Resources for Further Learning

Gain ideas and resources for ongoing and future work. The following resources have particular relevance in guiding clinical students.

- Team Strategies and Tools to Enhance Performance and Patient Safety (TeamSTEPPS). This is a federally sponsored, evidence-based program that teaches team communication, situation monitoring, leadership, and mutual support. www.ahrq.gov/teamstepps/index.html
- The Agency for Healthcare Research and Quality (AHRQ): This organization has an interesting variety of toolkits you or your students can explore (e.g., improved patient safety). AHRQ Quality and Patient Safety Programs www.ahrq.gov/programs/index.html?search_api_views_fulltext=&field_program_topics=14177

REFERENCES

American Association of Colleges of Nursing. (2008). The essentials of baccalaureate education for professional nursing practice. Retrieved from http://www.aacnnursing.org/Education-Resources/AACN-Essentials

American Nurses Association. (2013). *Patient handling and mobility: Interprofessional National Standards.* Silver Spring, MD: Author.

Benner, P., Kyriakidis, P., & Stannard, D. (2011). *Clinical wisdom and interventions in acute and critical care* (2nd ed.). New York, NY: Springer Publishing.

Berlinger, N. (2017). Workarounds Are Routinely Used by Nurses-But Are They Ethical? *American Journal of Nursing, 117*(10),53-55. doi:0.1097/01.NAJ.0000525875.82101.b7.

Bonnel, W., & Hober, C. (2016). Optimizing the reflective observer role in high-fidelity patient simulation. *Journal of Nursing Education,* 55(6):353–356. doi:10.3928/01484834-20160516-10

Erickson, J. I., Ditomassi, M., Sabia, S., & Smith, M. E. (2015). Creating a narrative culture. In J. Foster et al (Ed.), *Fostering clinical success: Using clinical narratives for interprofessional team partnerships. Massachusetts General Hospital.* Retrieved from http://www.reflectionsonnursingleadership.org/features/more-features/Vol41_2_creating-a-narrative-culture

Galloway, S. J. (2009). Simulation techniques to bridge the gap between novice and competent healthcare professionals. *Online Journal of Issues in Nursing, 14*(2), Manuscript 3. doi:10.3912/OJIN.Vol14No02Man03

Herrman, J. W. (2015). *Creative teaching strategies for the nurse educator*. Philadelphia, PA: F. A. Davis.

Hutchings, P., Ewell, P., & Banta, T. (2012). AAHE principles of good practice: Aging nicely. Retrieved from http://learningoutcomesassessment.org/PrinciplesofAssessment.html#AAHE

Institute of Medicine. (2008). Retooling for an aging America: Building the health care workforce. Retrieved from http://www.iom.edu/CMS/3809/40113/53452.aspx

Institute of Medicine Committee on the Health Professions Education. (2003). *Health professions education: A bridge to quality*. Washington, DC: National Academies Press.

Interprofessional Education Collaborative. (2016). *Core competencies for interprofessional collaborative practice: 2016 update*. Washington, DC. Retrieved from www.tamhsc.edu/ipe/research/ipec-2016-core-competencies.pdf

Lachman, V. D. (2015). Patient safety: The ethical imperative. Nursing world. Retrieved from http://www.nursingworld.org/MainMenuCategories/EthicsStandards/Resources/Patient-Safety.pdf

National League for Nursing. (2015). Debriefing across the curriculum. Retrieved from http://www.nln.org/docs/default-source/about/nln-vision-series-(position-statements)/nln-vision-debriefing-across-the-curriculum.pdf?sfvrsn=0

National League for Nursing. (2018). Advancing care excellence for seniors. Retrieved from http://www.nln.org/professional-development-programs/teaching-resources/ace-s

Quality and Safety Education for Nurses Institute. (2017). QSEN competencies. Retrieved from http://qsen.org/competencies

Squires, R. D. (2009). Electronic clinical logs. *Topics in Advanced Practice Nursing eJournal, 9*(3). Retrieved from https://www.medscape.com/viewarticle/708590

Thede, L., & Sewell, J. (2015). *Informatics and nursing: Competencies and applications*. Philadelphia, PA: Lippincott.

Walvoord, B. E., & Anderson, V. J. (2009). *Effective grading: A tool for learning and assessment in College*. San Francisco, CA: Jossey-Bass.

CHAPTER 15

Engaging Patients and Families for Safe, Quality Patient Care With Technology

CHAPTER GOAL

Gain perspective on the benefits and opportunities for engaging diverse patients and populations with technologies.

BEGINNING REFLECTION

What experiences have you had working with students to expand ways to use technologies in:

1. Expanding patient education for safe, quality care for patients and specific populations?
2. Enhancing assessment and planning for needs of specific communities and populations?
3. Engaging patients for safe, quality care in their home/community settings with tools such as telehealth?

Overheard: *I didn't know I had so many diabetic patients.*

Students want to understand their patients and populations to enhance their care approaches. Technologies can help expand learning and understanding for both. Patients can be considered experts on themselves and bring important information to the team. Patient education and technologies are concepts that take on increasing importance in healthcare for engaging patients as individuals and as people students will be caring for in their practices. Technologies follow them from acute to home settings as well.

Healthcare changes put more emphasis on patients using guided learning strategies to deal with acute/chronic health problems and manage lifestyle change and chronicity. Patients expect to be more informed care participants; a goal of patient education is to increase patient confidence and competence.

These concepts apply across settings and from chronic to acute care needs and issues. This chapter discusses opportunities for using technologies to engage patients and populations in health-promotion needs and the use of technologies such as telehealth in the home.

What Is Patient-Centered Care and What Does It Mean to Engage the Patient in Care? How Does Technology Help?

Patient-centered care and *engaged patient care* are two terms commonly used with different meanings. Naming what constitutes patient-centered care has been described as challenging by diverse entities. It includes listening to, informing, and involving patients in their care. In early work, the Institute of Medicine (IOM, 2001) described patient-centered care as care to patients that is respectful and responsive to patient needs, values, and preferences in patient care/decisions.

Engaged patient care involves the concept of the patient and family as part of the care team. Although clinicians provide scientific expertise, patients and families bring their personal knowledge of preferences and functional possibilities. Engaged patients are key components of a safe, effective healthcare system. Themes describing engagement (National Academy of Sciences [NAS], 2013) include patient engagement as a skill; health professionals need to listen fully, and culture dominates conversations (trust counts). It involves partnering with patients as full team members to drive shared decisions for better outcomes. Technology can help. Full toolkits using technology to guide patient engagement are available (e.g., the HIMSS patient engagement toolkit at *www .himss.org/library/patient-engagement-toolkit*).

It is important to guide students in building relevant engaging learning activities for patients. Patient education and health literacy concepts will be important tools for them to consider in their use of technology. Sample areas to focus students in engaging patients via technologies for education include the following:

- Keep the caring along with the technology. Do not let technology be a barrier to caring. Technologies can encourage patient and families to engage in their care, but balance high tech with high touch.
- Listen to the patient's story. Clinical conversations that address the patient's story help provide balance to a high-technology world. Knowing patients' stories help identify and engage patients in a plan that intertwines story with caring and technology. It provides an opportunity for patients to talk about their values and preferences, and for tough topics especially, it helps in getting their story. Story can lead to improved communication that helps providers and patients align treatment plans with patient values. Story also fits the health literacy topic. Consider education as having a conversation with the patient.
- Gain understanding of the patients' home setting and additional challenges that they may find in implementing treatment plans in their home

(a functional approach). For example, if working with an older adult with vision problems, the plan should include not only an understanding of medications and how to take them, but also include any functional issues with technology such as problems using visual devices for reminders or reading directions.

■ Pay attention to transition times such as hospital discharge. Patient education often occurs during transition times and typically includes conveying patient care plans to community based providers. Optimizing use of technologies such as EHRS can promote clear communication and minimize misunderstandings.

Patient Education and Technologies

Patients have been described as the underutilized resource in the patient care team. As patients assume more responsibility for their own care and well-being, one of the most important things nurses do to provide safety and quality care is patient education. Patient education in general provides opportunity for the provider to connect with patients on improving health goals. Patient education works best if providers know where the patient is and understand their story, knowledge level, and motivations. Technology promotes opportunities to help make this happen.

In nursing education, technology and patient education can serve to integrate many themes such as student cultural competence, patient health literacy, patient safety on the Internet, and common public health concerns. At a time of overflowing curriculum, gaining the most from online resources and broad concept-based assignments can be incorporated as strategies to integrate patient education concepts in an efficient way.

Patient education is more than providing patients with a handout. Patients, as well as students, need learning plans, as discussed in previous chapters. These plans may even work best when they involve technology as tool. Rather than just a class session on writing lesson plans, your students will need applied assignments to gain skills for good patient education. Much like faculty plan teaching (using their lesson plans to organize assessment, plans, implementation, and evaluation of student learning) students can learn to do this for their patients. In engaging students for good patient education, faculty help them build on what they know about best teaching and learning practices with technology. Points to help student recall include:

■ **Best-evidence resources are available.** Best practices such as "teach back" confirm understanding. Also, faculty should provide good, clearly communicated instructional materials for students to take home and should help students locate resources such as SPEAK UP for Patient Safety and Ask Me 3.

■ **Technology can support patient education.** This includes, for example, optimizing use of the web (rather than dealing with after effect problems). Other types of technology for patient education can also be engaged, including tools such as mobile devices and computers in waiting rooms, videos, online patient education texts, and email cues/reminders.

- **Technology and patient sensory issues need to be addressed.** Visual and auditory issues are particular concerns for aging adults. It is important that any technologies recommended to patients, such as mobile devices, have settings that allow adequate visibility including font size and color contrast. When using and communicating with patients via electronic health records, make sure to talk to the patient and not just the computer screen. Minimizing any background noise is also helpful.
- **The patient's story is important.** With the increasing use of technology, it is especially important to gain the patient's story to promote self-management. It is a conversation, setting the stage by understanding where patients are as a part of collaborating with them in the learning plan. In other words, it is a needs assessment.
- **Health literacy must be addressed.** Patient education is very clearly related to health literacy. This is especially important when working with patients from diverse cultures. Good patient education can help minimize communication errors for both the patient and the system.

Partnering With Patients for Web-Based Education

The Internet, presenting both opportunities and challenges in engaging patients, did not come with teaching instructions. With the advent of the Internet came a whole new way of thinking about patient education and the need to provide students guidance in help patients with safe healthy practices on the Internet. What can faculty do to help students partner with patients to be web savvy and promote responsible use of Internet resources? Sample ideas include:

- Assess patient needs. Students need to understand where their patients go for health information, including appropriate use of the Internet. Teach patients how to use websites more effectively. Build in opportunities for patients to ask follow-up questions, increasing their partnering with healthcare providers.
- Use the Internet to enhance, not replace, traditional patient education. This includes providing recommendations for good Internet resources patients can easily access and understand. Share, for example, sites that provide quality information and are useful to begin patient education resource lists; include respected sites such as National Institutes of Health (NIH) and national professional organizations.
- Make sure patients have good "pre-education" if they are searching the Internet on their own. Help patients learn to critique web resources when they search the Internet on their own (similar to students' guides

as discussed in Chapter 5) by providing critique guidelines for knowing a quality website with criteria such as credibility, content, disclosure, links, design, and interactivity.

Technology and Health Literacy Needs

Another important strategy for engaging students with patients is in promoting the use of good health literacy concepts. Health literacy, described as the ability to obtain the information that patients need to make reasonable health decisions, includes the degree to which patients can obtain, process, and understand basic health information and services (IOM, 2004). Patient self-management for healthcare then requires a patient's ability to navigate and communicate within the healthcare system. An adverse event is more likely to occur in state of poor health literacy (NAS, 2013). Some points to consider related to health literacy include:

- Students have limited impact on patients, healthcare systems, and public health without a focus on communication and health literacy concepts. Rather than thinking about this as additional content, it may be a way to focus many new important concepts within patient education assignments/discussions with students.
- Enhancing health literacy for patient education includes providing knowledge in easy to understand terms. This involves not only patient health related information, but can be as basic as direction finding in large healthcare organizations.
- Health literacy needs to be addressed in relation to culturally diverse patients. Traditional culture can be considered as shared ideas, meanings, and values with culture giving significance to health information and messages. A wide variety of social and cultural factors can lead to misinformation on health topics.

ENGAGING PATIENTS WITH PORTALS AND OTHER E-HEALTH RESOURCES

Patient Portals and Electronic Health Records

Patient portals are a summary of patients' data and reports in one healthcare system. Basically, they are a repository for patient data and might be considered serving as the patient's health story. Depending on the system, most e-health technologies can be used to monitor, track, and inform health decisions and to use digital technologies to enable health communication among practitioners and between health professionals and clients or patients. They are typically a component of the patient electronic health records and serve as tools to collect, manage, and use health data. The e-portal takes on increasing importance in care at home and with aging populations. There are benefits for the engaged patient and provider with a team focus. Although definitions vary, in general, e-portals differ from patient personal health records in a distinct way. Portals are owned and maintained by the healthcare system, whereas personal health records are owned and maintained by patients rather than their providers (often purchased or accessed via web resources). An interesting book called *Let Patients Help!* (deBronkart, 2013) provides further points from the patient perspective.

Appointment dates can be monitored, refills can be requested, clear communication can be gained for all about the dates, times, and places of care. Laboratory test results are easily monitored, and patterns even graphed (instead of having stacks of papers). Patients can benefit as they track presurgical and postsurgical appointments. Tracking of varied team appointments, such as physical therapy, along with system medical appointments, are tracked. Many also provide access to common patient questions/answers with generic information about basic diagnoses or treatments. The portal can help patient convey to their families the bigger picture or even to help monitor their care from a distance.

Patient Portals and Their Value

The value of patient portals includes helping to personalize a patient's health message; it is a useful repository for histories and record keeping. Patients have opportunity to check the accuracy of their data. Portals provide opportunities to record postdischarge communications from home and can help track patient problems or needs for further planning. They can promote self-management of chronic diseases and serve as reminder tools in primary prevention. Also, they can help patients' feel more like members of the healthcare team and help promote clear communication by all team members to avoid mistakes. Faculty can help students see the value of portals and the ways that they might be used, creating cases, for example, about their uses in chronic health management, such as diabetes or asthma, as well as more acute situations.

TECHNOLOGY TO ENGAGE PATIENTS FOR POPULATION HEALTH

Overview

Just as faculty emphasize to students the need for patient education for those with acute and chronic health problems, we also want to help patients in homes and communities to be proactive in approaches to their health. Promoting health and function in all populations makes sense for quality of life and healthcare system costs. Although traditional education models have had students focus primarily on individual patients, models such as the Quality and Safety Education for Nurses (QSEN) Institute extend thinking to focus on broad population and systems care.

Select Examples

The following examples will help faculty aid their students to think about technology as a tool for engaging their patients for health. Technology resources can be patient tools for gaining behavior prompts, motivators for promoting healthy behaviors, or monitoring of a chronic disease.

- **Adults and prompts for increasing activity.** The evidence supports, for example, that walking has multiple benefits, has little risk, and is relatively easy and cost effective. The big challenge is motivating people to start and maintain walking as an activity. Select technological strategies include exercise prompts, such as text messages and alarms, basic step counters linked to advanced pedometers, and special watches that monitor vitals, vary from health text messages and online social marketing (IOM, 2012).

- **Teens and apps for weight loss.** Although teens are at risk for challenges (such as stigma of being identified as overweight, emotional eating, and peer pressure) with weight management or weight loss, many have an interest in technology, which may help. Apps vary from self-assessment tools to recording individual activity patterns. They can help individuals gain needed nutritional details such as portion sizes, healthier food choices, and ways to read food labels.

- **Individuals and stress management.** The interplay of body, mind, and spirit are important for integrative health and wellness and is especially important in high-stress, high-tech healthcare settings. The NIH National Center for Complementary and Integrative Health collects best evidence on complementary approaches, which are summarized at their website (nccih.nih.gov). Web-based resources that guide health promotion include positive framing and complementary activities such as relaxation strategies and yoga. Apps exist for mind–body approaches, relevant for adding to daily routines for stress management for patients and others.

- **Older adults and safety tools.** Those dealing with challenges such as Alzheimer's disease can use apps/technologies to stay in their home. Examples can be shared about the potential for wearable technologies or home-monitoring devices to promote safety. Students can review evidence-based home safety resources from sources such as the Alzheimer's Association to gain further safety and technology ideas (www.alz.org/care/alzheimers-dementia-home-safety.asp).

- **Student health and web-based resources.** For example, using web-based resources, student can be guided in reviewing the overall Healthy People 2020 goals that include health promotion, health for all, optimal social and physical environment, and health behaviors for quality of life (U.S. Department of Health and Human Services, 2012). Assessments of educational programs can also be done to ensure that best evidence-based content on self-care and health behaviors are incorporated into the curriculum, with assignments that allow students to incorporate technology supports for their own self-care.

TECHNOLOGY TOOLS TO ASSESS AND PLAN FOR SPECIFIC COMMUNITY/POPULATION HEALTH NEEDS

Population health is an increasingly important focus in healthcare and a component of American Association of Colleges of Nursing (AACN, 2008) Essentials. Technologies, often considered in relation to individuals' health needs. For example, studying disaster preparedness in community or population health courses, students learn about tools for knowledge access (such as community health risk assessments, disaster planning, communication, and dissemination) as well as using evidence-based protocols to improve response readiness. Students can gain additional experience using technology for population need assessment and planning.

Population Need Assessments

A population focus in health promotion includes building on available resources and working with people in their communities to promote health. Population health issues vary by setting and population, so faculty should guide students in using technology to generate need assessments to better understand specific, unique populations. Sample opportunities for considering technology in expanding the traditional tools of document reviews, observations, and informal interviews include the following.

- Use available Internet resources and documents to review and analyze population needs. This can include data collection for local, state, and national data repositories to gain information on specific populations (i.e., stroke rates in local, state, and national repositories).
- Consider community "place" factors. Students, often without leaving their desks, can use technologies to observe and gain a broader context and perspective. What technologies are helpful in describing community place factors? Examples include Google Earth and GPS systems.
- Consider audio/video conferencing interview opportunities and electronic surveys as ways to gain additional data from community members.

Planning for Population Needs

Once students complete need assessments, they can analyze and identify community needs and strengths to set the stage for further work, creating projects with technology for populations based on needs. Ask students to brainstorm how technologies could best help with the following potential projects:

- Identify gaps and create technology-based projects to strengthen resources (e.g., resource directories to benefit informal home caregivers or primary care offices).

- Build on available informal and formal community networks and resources, emphasizing their positive resources.
- Partner with families and local community agencies to develop creative health programs such as smoking cessation or weight loss, delivered in connection with local churches or other organizations using technology resources.
- Work with community-based primary care settings to identify needed educational resources. Help to develop evidence-based resources for select problems, including teaching protocols (using technology to create best-communication messages).
- Generate health information products such as simple brochures with technology to communicate to multiple groups.

ENGAGING PATIENTS WITH TECHNOLOGY IN THE HOME TO PROMOTE PATIENT SAFETY AND QUALITY CARE

Although community health nursing has long been a curriculum staple, less emphasis has been on home nursing and clinician care relationships in that setting. Technologies bring new opportunities including telehealth and even expanded phone nursing.

Helping Students Help Patients and Their Families Prepare for Using Technology in Their Homes

How can technology tools help engage patients for safe, quality care in their home/community settings? When home becomes the healthcare setting, what do all need to know about technologies and/or telehealth? The following section on technologies in the home and telehealth provides concepts and sample assignments to guide student learning needs related to patients with chronic care needs, newly transitioning patients, and those requiring mental healthcare.

How are patients and families best prepared to use technology? Patient are often discharged from the hospital after acute illnesses to manage ongoing care needs on their own (sometimes this involves family helpers and sometimes not). After an older adults' acute pneumonia and need for home health monitoring following hospitalization, for example, an array of technologies may be delivered to the home for monitoring vitals, weight, oxygen saturations, and other parameters. These health-management devices, sensors, and even activity monitors provide students opportunities to learn about biometric medical devices, such as pulse oximetry, and peak flow meters as they help families learn about using these tools. How are patients/families best prepared to participate with this care, especially with an accompanying illness challenge? Good patient orientation to the technologies is indicated, extending beyond just dropping off the equipment. Phone follow-up opportunities are needed as well.

Preparing Students for Technologies in the Home—Telehealth

Learning about telehealth continues students' opportunities to participate in improving patient care in the home. Students need to be prepared to participate in this changing approach to healthcare, gaining skills in monitoring, and supporting patients at a distance.

Telehealth serves as tool to improve connections with patients at a distance. It involves the remote delivery of healthcare services and involves various communication technologies and incorporates nursing practice/engagement of a patient at a remote site. The interaction includes reviewing health status, treatment plans, and monitoring of responses and outcomes (National Council of State Boards of Nursing, 2014). There are varied concepts and descriptors of telehealth, and consistent with other technologies, the boundaries are blurring. Telehealth is described as including the collection of clinical data for disease management, providing disease-prevention programs, real-time video for emergent care needs, and follow-up healthcare services. Healthcare services are delivered, managed, and coordinated by nurses and other health providers.

Telehealth involves understanding pathways and protocols. As people seek care in their home settings versus more structured care facilities, students learn that new technologies make this care more possible. Telehealth does not seem foreign if one considers that telehealth is at least as old as telephone advice. Phone advice services provided by urgent care health professionals or phone follow-up by a nurse from a physician's office are familiar approaches.

A technology champion, Katie Crossland, describes her rural hospital leadership role, engaging rural staff in implementing a telehealth program for diverse patients at a distance. She provides an overview of issues for student and staff development in implementing rural telehealth, describing not only challenges, but also creative solutions, to addressing problems with this major undertaking (Exhibit 15.1).

Telehealth as an Extension of Traditional Phone Nursing

Phone nursing, long in use, provides commonsense approaches for helping patients cope with acute or chronic problems. There are benefits in teaching students about phone nursing because it can help improve the connection factor. Conversations with providers and clients provide a human interface to balance high-tech healthcare systems. Nurses encourage patients, provide guidance, and answer questions. Phone connections can help patients with self-management goals to increase their confidence and care abilities.

The case management role and phone nursing are one of the more recent developments, especially in models for individuals dealing with chronic disease such as congestive heart failure and diabetes. Other phone nurse roles include

EXHIBIT 15.1

FACULTY CHAMPION: RURAL TELEHEALTH TIPS

Katie Crossland, MSN, RN

1. *What is your current position like, relevant to implementing rural telehealth?* As Director of Nursing in our facility, I have had to help implement telehealth into our Emergency and Acute Care departments. Part of the process included training our staff when to use the telehealth resource and then also how to use it. Our facility also uses telehealth in our outpatient department with pulmonology and mental health. We continue to look for additional opportunities to bring additional telehealth services to the people of our community and surrounding area.

2. *What formal or informal education or training you have had in rural telehealth?* My initial education with a rural facility was on-the-job training from other experienced nurses. When we implemented our emergency department and acute care telehealth resource at the facility where I work, I was already comfortable in using telehealth, so my training was not extensive but just an overview of how the system worked and needed to be maintained. We continue to have an update on use of the telehealth resource once a year as a refresher course in the use of the system.

3. *What ways do you see staff benefiting from better understanding of rural telehealth?* Telehealth is the way of the future for rural hospitals. With it becoming more difficult to recruit providers to rural America, telehealth allows the population to seek advanced services at the convenience of their local facility. Understanding and being comfortable with using telehealth services not only makes the nurses' job easier, but also helps make the patient's experience positive.

4. *What are some of the strategies you use in engaging rural staff with technologies?* Technology is either an exciting or a scary concept to nursing staff, often depending on their age, with younger staff typically more enthusiastic. Education about the equipment is key in implementing telehealth or new equipment. If the leader stays excited about the technology and shows the benefits it will have for patients and staff, then the buy-in from staff will be enhanced. The other tactic that helps staff better understand the technology and its benefits is using it. Once they gain hands-on experience and reap the benefits for themselves and their patients, the willingness to use the technology drastically increases.

5. *What are key point's nurse educator students need to better understand related to teaching and learning needs with technology in the rural setting?* Make sure your students understand how rural medicine is changing and how telehealth helps keep the doors of the critical access hospitals open. Students need to have an understanding of computer and iPad use and must understand HIPAA and ways to keep personal health information secure when using such technology. Along with that, they need to understand that in rural facilities, you may wear multiple hats and therefore may be the nurse for the patient and the IT department if you have any difficulties with the technology.

6. *What are select facilitators for incorporating rural telehealth into staff development or nursing education courses/programs?* Educating the staff and getting them to use the equipment on a regular basis helps develop them into proficient users of telehealth. When incorporating rural telehealth into student courses, keep the information up to date, and visit facilities that use telehealth so that you can understand

(continued)

the fundamentals and the way it affects nursing operations. Have nursing staff from rural facilities visit your classes to discuss their experiences. Technology is changing the way nursing is done in general, so when you discuss technology in your classes, telehealth could be a portion of that discussion.

7. *What are some of the challenges of incorporating rural telehealth into staff development or nursing education courses/programs?* The change factor is the biggest challenge we face. Staff may be reluctant to use a technology in which the person we are speaking to or the provider giving orders is not standing in the room next to you but may be multiple states away. Then there is the fact of technology. Some people are not technologically savvy and therefore shy away from any use of it, thereby making it difficult to properly use telehealth services. Personal attitudes toward telehealth can also be a barrier. If the nurse is not comfortable with telehealth, that feeling can be relayed to patients, who then will not have the positive experience that telehealth really can provide.

8. *In what ways do you work with interprofessional colleagues in rural telehealth?* Telehealth gives us the ability to work with different disciplines a majority of the time. We can have providers, specialty nurses, and pharmacists working together on the same patient simultaneously. Along with that, staff with the patient are the eyes and ears for the provider on the other side of the screen, giving them important information that can change of the course of treatment for the patient. Telehealth provides a great interprofessional approach to healthcare for our patients.

9. *What tips or advice would you like to share with new educators teaching about rural telehealth?* Rural nursing is one of the many diverse opportunities of the profession. Telehealth will continue to affect the way rural medicine/nursing is performed. With that being said, faculty should teach the importance of adaptability to technology in the rural setting. As noted, make sure to teach the importance of HIPAA and keeping health information secure as we live in a litigation-prone generation. Another aspect of the rural setting is that telehealth will help keep the doors of our critical access hospitals open by keeping patients coming in the doors and not having to drive hours to see a specialty provider.

HIPAA, Health Insurance Portability and Accountability Act.

management of information needs in primary care and after-hour clinic phone needs. Students can learn to assess and plan with standardized tools typically used in formal phone nursing programs. There is value in using structured assessment and follow-up protocols to help keep all team members aware of the information documented and the recommended follow-up plans. Phone nursing ideally is combined with EHRS and patient portal resources to promote consistency of information.

Preparing Students to Care for Patients Via Telehealth

Extending phone nurse abilities with telehealth technology can allow patient assessment data such as heart and lung sounds to be transmitted electronically to specialty providers. Digital images such as x-rays or photos of skin lesions can be transmitted. Given the appropriate technology, healthcare providers can connect with patients and families in their homes for routine check-ins and electronic reminders. Sample skills needed in telehealth nursing include both technological and interpersonal skills, practice knowledge, and administrative skills, including documentation and resource management.

Students can gain skills for assisting patients in their home setting as faculty prepare students to use technologies in monitoring and providing care at a distance. With the aging population, for example, there are benefits in learning about tools to help older adults remain in their homes. Faculty can ask students to read, review Internet resources, and think creatively about how technologies can enhance safety and life quality for individuals choosing to remain at home. Telehealth provides clinical opportunities for students learning from home settings to rural clinics and caregivers.

One example for preparing students in the mental health field for telehealth is provided by Dr. Martha Baird. Dr. Baird learned from personal teaching experiences about the importance of focusing on telehealth teaching strategies specific to mental health nursing. Here work with students led to program development and increased quality work for her graduates who will be working with patients at a distance. Further discussion is provided in Exhibit 15.2.

EXHIBIT 15.2

TIPS FROM FACULTY CHAMPIONS: TELEHEALTH TEACHING APPROACHES FOR MENTAL HEALTH CLINICIANS

Martha B. Baird, PhD, APRN/CNS-BC, CTN-A

Telemental health (TMH) is the use of live, interactive videoconference (VC) for the purpose of delivery of mental health and substance abuse services from one geographic location to another (National Institute of Mental Health [2010]). TMH is considered an acceptable, effective, and efficient method for providing psychiatric services to diverse populations such as children, the elderly, and the disabled. TMH provides services for those with limited access to mental health services such those living in rural areas, prisons, and residential treatment centers. An online survey conducted by the author revealed that a majority of PMH-APRNs have used TMH in the delivery of psychiatric services with their patients, yet few reported any formal education or training in this delivery method (Baird, Whitney, & Caedo, 2017).

The NLN (2016) has set a priority to build the science of nursing education through the discovery and translation of innovative evidence-based strategies using technology, simulation, and virtual experiences to enhance student learning that affects clinical practice. In response to this call, we developed evidence-based TMH educational guidelines for PMH-APRN students. Students enrolled in a graduate PMH-APRN practitioner program at a large U.S. university in the Midwest were educated about the principles of TMH delivery methods.

In our psychiatric PMH-APRN program, we have used SPs (actors trained to enact the role of a patient with a scripted mental condition) to simulate patient encounters in two of the core courses, advanced psychiatric assessment and the final practicum.

(continued)

Until a few years ago, these simulated encounters were conducted in-person in a laboratory set up as a primary clinic setting, which included a desktop computer and a video camera. The SP encounters are video recorded, and the SP provides verbal feedback to each student at the conclusion. Students view their own video-recorded interview and complete a series of self-assessments. The faculty then reviews the video-recorded student/SP encounter and provides written feedback to each student.

When our PMH-APRN program transitioned to an online format in the summer of 2014, we began offering the simulated SP experience using telemonitors. At this point, we realized that students were not adequately prepared to use this video-conferencing format and that we needed to educate them about TMH delivery methods, in addition to the skills of conducting a psychiatric assessment.

We received feedback from our faculty, technicians, and the SPs, all of whom noted that students needed training in TMH delivery methods. It was apparent that the principles of professionalism, confidentiality, and a professional practice environment for the online encounters were not being translated. We introduced an online lecture about the basic principles of TMH delivery and required each student to have an individual session with a technician prior to the SP encounter to provide direction and coaching about computer connectivity, encryption for patient privacy, professional dress, and setup of a work environment. Follow-up module topics include telemental health, ethical/legal issues, licensure/coding/billing, interprofessional collaboration, and safety concerns.

Nurses are at the forefront of addressing the mental health needs of populations. Therefore, it is essential that PMH-APNs be adequately prepared in this innovative and rapidly expanding practice delivery method.

NLN, National League for Nursing; PMH-APRN, psychiatric mental health advanced practice nurse; SP, standardized patient; TMH, telemental health; VC, videoconferencing.

Broad telehealth examples for creating assignments include the following:

- Inviting practicing telehealth clinicians to the classroom
- Interviewing or observing participants
- Monitoring a patient with a chronic illness in the home and considering best technology uses
- Working with clinicians in a clinical rotation to provide off-site care monitoring
- Treating schoolchildren with illness in partnership with a school nurse

Selected organizations providing further information on telehealth include the following:

- American Telemedicine Association: www.americantelemed.org
- American Academy of Ambulatory Care Nursing (AAACN): www.aaacn.org
- Office for the Advancement of Telehealth: www.hrsa.gov/rural-health/telehealth/index.html

SUMMARY

Patient education, technology, and telehealth are concepts that take on increasing importance in healthcare because patients are encouraged to engage in their care. A focus on population healthcare is also increasing. New and emerging technologies help extend caregiving resources to the home and community settings.

ENDING REFLECTIONS FOR YOUR LEARNING NOTEBOOK

1. What is the most important content that you learned in this chapter?
2. What are your plans for using the information provided in this chapter in your future teaching endeavors?
3. What are your further learning goals?

GUIDELINES FOR TEACHING AND LEARNING WITH TECHNOLOGIES

Quick Teaching Tips

1. Focus students on thinking how they engage technologies in their clinical work, emphasizing caring approaches to help with rapport.
2. Revisit patient education in your curriculum. What ways can patient education assignments be integrated with other content, including health literacy concepts.
3. Think population health—consider how community health and population assignments can be enhanced with technologies.

Questions for Further Reflection

1. What are your roles and responsibilities related to engaging future students to promote patients' safe, quality care with technology? Can you identify ways to incorporate student learning on the following?
   - Identify technology tools for patient education that uses best evidence and that incorporate health literacy considerations.
   - Use technology tools that expand patient education for specific population needs (health promotion needs; online risk assessments). Determine which education tools (web resources, apps) can also be used.
   - Use technology tools that expand assessment and planning for the needs of specific communities and populations.
2. Engage patients for safe, quality care in their home or community setting?

LEARNING ACTIVITY: DEVELOPING ASSIGNMENTS FOR YOUR STUDENTS

Choose from the following to create assignments for your current or future students. The purpose of this activity is to help think about diverse technology opportunities with diverse patients.

- **Web education:** What is right about the Internet and current approaches for patient education? What are challenges? What case examples (positive or negative) and lessons learned can you share from your experiences?
- **Health literacy and patient engagement:** Review the HIMSS site for patient engagement strategies (www.himss.org/library/patient-engagement -toolkit). How could you use the following resources to engage patients in their care?
  - Wearables and mobile apps
  - Social media and online patient communities

ONLINE RESOURCES FOR FURTHER LEARNING

This resource review can help you gain ideas and resources for ongoing and future work. The following have particular reference in guiding your students in engaging patients and populations for health promotion.

- HIMSS Patient Engagement. www.himss.org/library/patient-engagement -toolkit
- Healthy People 2020. www.healthypeople.gov/2020/topics-objectives
- Communicating to Advance the Public's Health. www.nap.edu/catalog/ 21694/communicating-to-advance-the-publics-health-workshop -summary
- Office for the Advancement of Telehealth. www.cchpca.org/office -advancement-telehealth-oat

REFERENCES

American Association of Colleges of Nursing. (2008). The essentials of baccalaureate education for professional nursing practice. Retrieved from http://www.aacnnursing.org/Education-Resources/ AACN-Essentials

Baird, M. B., Whitney, L., & Caedo, C. E. (2017). Experiences and attitudes among psychiatric mental health advanced practice nurses in the use of telemental health: Results of an online survey. *Journal of the American Psychiatric Nurses Association*. Advance online publication. doi:10.1177/1078390317717330

deBronkart, D. (2013). *Let patients help!* Seattle, WA: CreateSpace Independent Publishing Platform.

Institute of Medicine. (2004). Health literacy: A prescription to end confusion. Retrieved from https:// www.nap.edu/catalog/10883/health-literacy-a-prescription-to-end-confusion

Institute of Medicine. (2012). *Accelerating progress in obesity prevention: Solving the weight of the nation*. Washington, DC: National Academies Press.

Kobylarz, F. A., Pomidor, A., & Heath, J. M. (2006). SPEAK. A mnemonic tool for addressing health literacy concerns in geriatric clinical encounters. *Geriatrics, 61*(7), 20–26.

National Academy of Sciences. (2013). Organizational change to improve health literacy: Workshop summary. Retrieved from http://nationalacademies.org/hmd/reports/2013/organizational-change-to-improve-health-literacy.aspx

National Council of State Boards of Nursing. (2014). The National Council of State Boards of Nursing position paper on the telehealth nursing practice. Retrieved from https://www.ncsbn.org/14_Telehealth.pdf

National Institute of Mental Health. (2010). Global leading categories of diseases/disorders (YLDs). Retrieved from https://www.nimh.nih.gov/health/statistics/global/global-leading-categories-of-diseases-disorders-ylds.shtml

National League for Nursing. (2016). NLN research priorities in nursing education 2016–2019. Retrieved from http://www.nln.org/professional-development-programs/research/research-priorities-in-nursing-education

CHAPTER 16

Special Contexts for Educational Leadership With Technology

CHAPTER GOAL

Explore leader/mentor/champion roles with technology in nursing education programs.

BEGINNING REFLECTION

1. What experiences have you had with leading or mentoring faculty development in using and applying technologies?
2. What experiences have you had with the leader/mentor role with integrating technologies into the curriculum?
3. What experiences have you had with opportunities for partnering in diverse teaching and learning contexts, such as staff development, with shared resources?

Overheard: *No one seems to want to change the curriculum. How are we supposed to make this happen?*

The leader or technology champion takes on many roles. These include mentoring others on technology, integrating technology into curriculum, and considering special contexts for using technologies. This chapter is about engaging and mentoring faculty and clinical team members. It includes taking the teaching and learning concepts reviewed earlier in the text and expanding them to work with diverse students and colleagues across diverse settings. In this chapter, select roles of leading and mentoring, curriculum leadership, and leadership opportunities for partnering and teaching and learning in diverse contexts are considered. Quality improvement (QI) concepts and technology as tools to help are emphasized.

LEADERSHIP AND MENTORING ROLES WITH AND FOR TECHNOLOGY

To keep up with rapid changes in healthcare and technologies, all faculty and their graduates need leadership and mentoring skills. Although the complexity of the healthcare system is often addressed in the literature, there is limited focus on the additional mentoring needs. Often, this task of engaging the team falls to new clinical educators. Guidance for coaching other team members and gaining situation context are key foci. All teachers are leaders. As many faculty have had few role models for teaching with technology, a steep learning curve exists without a mentor to guide us. Trusted teaching and learning principles and theories serve in guiding work, but mentors, as trusted counselors, also champion our work with technology. Learning about rapidly emerging technology often involves finding champions of specific technology approaches and learning from these mentors.

Throughout this text, champion exhibits provide examples of mentoring and leadership. Gaining a mentor who is willing to share teaching tips or conversation on selected teaching with technology projects can enhance our work. Basic facilitating tips that can guide are discussed in the following paragraphs.

Mentoring for Faculty Development

Mentoring definitions vary, but in general, it is considered a guided experience, facilitating development and seeking success outcomes as defined by the discipline and/or setting. It is an approach to engage and motivate our mentees and includes support from an experienced individual. Its aim is to guide mentees on journey of clinical learning, including information, encouragement, and role modeling.

Other related terms include *coaching, role modeling, precepting*, and *teaching*. Often, it is considered on a spectrum moving from a formal program to informal situational mentoring. Best practices in mentoring can promote optimal use of time as well as improved outcomes. We want to clarify our roles, identify resources to guide us, and consider our goals. Educational leaders will have ultimate goals of recruiting, retaining, and strengthening the profession.

Being a mentor includes recognizing the creativity of faculty and staff, both new and experienced. Although mentoring is often considered with new, or transitioning faculty, it is also important to address the needs of adjuncts and new clinical faculty. These individuals are sometimes forgotten with new processes/technologies.

Common principles and useful mentoring tools include the following:

1. Understand your role as mentor: Self-reflect—what is your perspective? What has worked/not worked when you mentored, or were mentored by others?
2. Learn about mentees: What is their background? Their perspectives on the situation? Hopes and goals?
3. Share via motivation, time, talent, and resources: Alternate coaching and cheerleading roles.

4. Provide a safe environment for staff and use a pattern of listening, coaching, guiding, and mentoring.
5. Devise good communication models, including skillful listening, powerful questions, and affirmation and challenges (feedback).
6. Give feedback that offers support and encouragement, providing direction and uses the opportunity to reflect on further opportunities.
7. Use reflective strategies (i.e., reflection, motivational self-talk, reflective logs, journals). Reflection as a tool of mentors allows opportunity to step back, take a deep breath, and process one's facts and reactions. The mentor/facilitator can help process thoughts when things are difficult and help keep the big picture in perspective.
8. Create accountability: Include meetings with action agendas (who, what, when), meeting summaries, and action items.

Help Mentees Put Learning/Action Plans Together

Mentees, along with their mentor, can assess gaps relevant to specific goals. This can include, for example, looking at standards that the mentee is aspiring to (such as National League for Nursing [NLN] educator competencies) and assessing gaps and need. Mentees, along with their mentor, can then set goals for making further action plans. Background for this work includes

- Help learners to identify goals, identify a plan, and provide support and feedback.
- Help learners stay focused on their goals/encourage support via progress/challenges.
- Help your mentee network and develop professional relationships. Identify informal to formal professional development opportunities, including, but not limited to, involvement in professional organizations.

Guide Your Mentee in Gaining Needed Resources

Mentors should guide mentees to specific resources such as relevant textbooks and online resources. They should ask whether needed courses or workshops are readily available. Are there webinars or seminars to gain new technologies information? If not, what alternatives can be addressed? A mentor/champion helps faculty find specific resources such as the following:

- Advancing Care Excellence for Seniors (ACES): NLN.
- Simulation Innovation Resource Center (SIRC): The NLN simulation center (sirc.nln.org). This site provides resources and ongoing discussion board topics.
- Quality and Safety Education for Nurses (QSEN) Institute: Based on the Institute of Medicine (IOM) Health Professions Educator Competencies, the QSEN Institute has developed objectives and resources to guide teaching and learning in these domains.

Additionally, mentees have responsibility to optimize their mentee role. Further tips for having a successful mentoring experience, such as being clear on goals and commitment to a working relationship, are shared by Phillips and Denison (2015).

Informal and Peer Mentoring With Technologies

Options for mentoring also include informal mentoring opportunities and peer colleague mentoring. Information about informal mentoring, for example, can be gained from the literature, following the works of experts in our technology area of interest. Often text authors provide additional journal articles or online resources for review. Additionally, peer colleagues can serve a supportive and encouraging function as local faculty members become learning partners in working on a technology project together. Developing a peer group of technology champions can also promote enthusiasm and creativity in developing course projects. Tools such as the New Technology Readiness Inventory (Exhibit 1.2) and the Integrated Learning Triangle for Teaching With Technologies (Exhibit 1.3) can provide direction.

Technology provides new ways of mentoring such as distance mentoring and electronic journal clubs. While we now have easy access to mentors and peer colleagues at a distance, just as with local mentors, being respectful of a mentor's time is important. Having a plan or agenda helps the team identify what is needed in an online meeting, what the goals and evaluation plans are, and how follow-up meetings will be scheduled. Finding a mentor at a distance is often facilitated by national programs such as the Sigma Theta Tau and NLN mentoring programs. Both programs serve as examples of mentoring at a national level in which prominent individuals provide guidance in selected project work. Further guides are available with tips for setting up mentoring plans, both as a mentor and as a mentee (NLN, 2006; Zachary, 2000).

CURRICULUM LEADERSHIP AND TECHNOLOGY (NURSING INFORMATICS EXAMPLE)

Overview

Technology, curriculum, and leadership are concepts that fit well together. Faculty leaders or champions bring knowledge and resources to the faculty/ curricula table. Aware of big-picture organization requirements (and how the internal system works), they meet faculty at the curriculum table to identify best approaches for a given program. The mentoring role continues related to curriculum as addressed in this section.

As you learn about new technologies and informatics concepts relevant to your educator role, it will be important for you to engage faculty colleagues in discussions on the value of these concepts or strategies for your curriculum. Curriculum helps in thinking beyond individual student to broad program-level outcomes. It is also one of the NLN educator competencies. Champions/leaders need to understand how curriculum processes work in their program as they consider technology projects or content/courses. This type of QI is as much about assessment and reflection as components of curriculum review and/or development. As leaders in QI and guiding students in care of patients, faculty can review the curriculum to provide an opportunity to critique and think about current processes for engaging students to become safe/quality clinicians with technology.

What Is Meant By Curriculum?

It is not just about the one session or one course that you teach, but the context and totality of student learning—you are going for. It brings us back to the Integrated Learning Triangle for Teaching With Technologies. It is part of naming what we do. Good concept descriptors are important in curriculum work. These concept descriptors are best when they provide program guidance and can be adapted to diverse contexts within the program. The following project exemplar provides guidance related to nursing informatics.

If your technology interest is nursing informatics (NI), for example, you may learn from others' work. What is the status of NI-related concepts in your curriculum? As summarized by Larson (2017) in a study addressing NI issues in nursing curricula, she learned about needs for assessing and planning for NI in curricula, as well as challenges and strategies in addressing these needs and issues. She found that basic staff development; technology, equipment, and resources; and ways to locate them influenced the integration of NI. To help address challenges, the leader/mentor asks the following questions: Where is NI currently and how will we know it is needed or wanted? The goal is to focus on identifying the "what is" of a current program and determining the "what is desired" in a future program (while keeping in mind internal and external forces that influence). Dr. Lisa Larson completed a dissertation gaining descriptive information from a statewide sample of faculty leaders who are engaged in implementing NI into the curriculum. Pleasantly surprised about their enthusiasm, she also learned about their challenges. Larson shares her leadership experiences related to the importance of NI to the curriculum in Exhibit 16.1.

EXHIBIT 16.1

TIPS FROM CHAMPIONS: BETTER UNDERSTANDING NURSING INFORMATICS IN NURSING PROGRAMS

Lisa Larson, PhD, RN

1. ***What is your current position, and what responsibilities related to NI are a part of your position?*** As an assistant dean in a baccalaureate nursing program, I find competency in NI as imperative to effectively function in contemporary, technology-rich, and information-saturated healthcare settings. One of my responsibilities is to see that nursing faculty have the NI knowledge, skills, and resources necessary to prepare

(continued)

students competent in NI knowledge and skills. In addition, I am responsible for see-ing that NI is adequately integrated in classroom and clinical experiences.

2. ***What formal or informal education or training have you had in NI, and how does it sup-port your current position?*** I received formal education in NI in my PhD program, completing a 21-credit minor in NI. In addition, my dissertation work focused on the perspectives and experiences of BSN program leaders related to NI in the cur-riculum (Larson, 2017). This education enabled me to accurately understand the purpose of NI and its importance and relationship with patient care and nursing education. I am able to serve as a resource to faculty and emphasize the impor-tance of NI in educating new nurses that will be responsible for managing patient health information using multiple kinds of HIT.

3. ***What are some of the issues you find related to NI and schools of nursing specific to the continuity of learning from the educational setting to clinical practice settings?*** Accurate, quality documentation of patient health information in a patient's health record is an important student skill. However, the availability and adequacy of tech-nology resources in the educational setting are major challenges. For example, the cost of a simulated EHR, also called an *academic EHR*, may be prohibitive. Even the more sophisticated academic EHRs may not be able to perform some functions of a "real" EHR. Also, differences among health information systems and restricted student access in clinical settings pose challenges to student learning. Finally, for a variety of reasons, faculty in nursing programs may find it difficult to remain current with rapidly changing and increasingly complex HIT.

4. ***What are the key points nurse educator students need to understand related to NI and teaching and learning issues in nursing programs? Why is this important to understand?*** The focus of NI is information, not technology. Technology is simply the tool used to manage health information. The goal of using HIT is improved patient safety, patient outcomes, and quality of care. Helping students understand these goals creates rele-vancy for learning and applying NI content and skills. For example, engaging students with patient health data in a quality-improvement project demonstrates the value of NI. In addition, a faculty champion for NI is a key resource. A faculty champion is a resource for the knowledge, skills, and attitudes needed by faculty to successfully integrate NI into the curriculum and demonstrate its value to students.

5. ***What are some challenges of using NI assignments to engage individuals on select topics? What recommendations do programs have for ongoing needs/work?*** Again, helping stu-dents see the relevancy of the assignment to clinical practice is key. Otherwise, they may dismiss learning NI concepts or skills as unimportant. In general, the younger generation is more familiar and comfortable with using technology, but there are wide skill sets between learners. Beginning students sometimes find identifying important pieces of information or prioritizing information difficult because they are still learning basic nursing knowledge and skills. Strengthening students' critical thinking skills is essential to preparing them for the complexities of patient care.

6. ***What advice would you like to share with new or future nurse educators about what you have learned about integrating NI into nursing programs?*** Faculty leaders and cham-pions can provide useful resources such as the QSEN competencies. Also, nurse educators need a common understanding of NI and consensus on what knowledge and skills are requisite for student learning in their programs. Students need to see the relevancy of learning activities in the educational environment to the clinical practice environment. In addition, nurse educators need the support of program leaders for providing instructional resources and faculty-development opportunities for keeping current with NI skills. Access to an NI expert or faculty champion can be key support resources.

EHR, electronic health record; HIT, health information technology; NI, nursing informatics; QSEN, Quality and Safety Education for Nurses (Institute).

Completing a Curriculum Needs Assessment

To further address NI (or other topical areas for curriculum), it is important to consider and know that a potential course or content integration is needed. Curriculum leaders can complete needs assessments (a type of gap analysis) of new/needed content in the curriculum. Curriculum points to consider in preparation for assessing/planning include the following:

- **Complete a thorough review** of the literature on curriculum topics.
- **Review important documents** relevant to your curriculum interest. Summarize recommendations for needed NI content such as that documented in the American Association of Colleges of Nursing (AACN) Essentials and The Joint Commission clinical guides. Use guidelines provided by national nursing organizations/other major resources to help identify critical content for courses/programs.
- **Review program context** and complete a needs assessment. What is currently there? This might begin by considering where the desired content might be covered to some degree in current program courses. What does a review of the current objectives for existing courses show?
- **Engage vested parties** in sharing needed curriculum perspectives. Gain additional input/perspectives on needs from stakeholders in curriculum such as students, service providers, and community members.

Creating a Course or Plan for Integrating Content

Once curriculum leaders have a complete need assessments and determined that there is a need for new or expanded content in the curriculum, they begin to lead the organization of a plan. The following are sample strategies. Think how you might address NI content in your designated curriculum:

- **Consider the Integrated Learning Triangle for Teaching With Technologies:** Once course planning begins, remember to consider the Integrated Learning Triangle for Teaching With Technologies and think about how content/learning activities and evaluation flow from course objectives and from program objectives. Use mind maps or concept maps to help get the course planning process started.
- **Map it out:** Try to visualize the end product for your curriculum project as you begin. For example, what competencies should your graduates have with NI? Will new content be integrated across the curriculum? Or addressed in one specific course?
- **Consider resources:** What resources, such as faculty expertise, faculty development, and technology resources will be needed? How will they be addressed? What are the costs of incorporating this course or program into the curriculum? Can available resources be used to meet this need? How are similar schools handling this issue?
- **Identify Policies:** For the changes they plan, leaders need to have policies in place and monitor their use. For example, with informatics

content, major faculty concerns often relate to potential legal and ethical issues related to student access and use of data.

- **Consider course clinical (or applied) components:** Are clinical agencies available for a clinical component? Are academic/agency partners set up to work with your students?
- **Plan for evaluation:** Consistent with ongoing QI, the goal is good program outcomes. Build in an evaluation plan that considers curriculum change, such as new NI content, and address how the NI learning activities and outcomes will be evaluated. In naming outcomes, consider the potential impact of your curriculum change on both individuals and the community.
- **Address the change process and system pathways:** Within your organization consider potential driving and restraining forces relevant to your curriculum change. Outline a plan that engages faculty, staff, and students for the change.

Developing a Course/Program Proposal (or New Technology Proposal)

Once needs and a tentative plan are identified for new informatics or technology related content, a proposal helps document the plan to clarify numerous considerations. A proposal, for example, can help you prepare for a presentation to your program's curriculum committee. The following questions can serve as a type of checklist to see if you have addressed major factors.

1. Why is the course important? Why does the learner need this information? Is there general support for specific course content (i.e., support from the local community, recommendations from a national association, review of the evidence-based literature)?
2. How will the course interface with the school curriculum/program framework, as well as be consistent with the school/university mission, philosophy, general education requirements?
3. How will the course author capture the "must-know" content? What textbook and specific teaching strategies will be appropriate for meeting course objectives? How will the teaching strategies measure up against current standards and best practices?
4. What, if any, unique considerations exist with the particular students who will likely take this course (i.e., student level, adequate prerequisites)?
5. Are aspects of the course relationship to the external environment addressed? For example, will students work with an external agency for a clinical component of the course?
6. What student evaluative outcomes will the course or program lead to? How will the course support achievement of total program outcomes/competencies?
7. What accrediting agency is used by your program (i.e., NLN, AACN)? Is the course consistent with any accreditation and/or regulatory requirements? Have you considered content guidance from national

resources such as the QSEN Institute's or other important professional documents?

8. Have you confirmed the correct agency that accredits your program?
9. Does the proposal also include a syllabus that operationalizes the plan? This includes the course objective, content outline, learning activities, and evaluation plan.

LEADERSHIP AND CLINICAL PARTNERING IN DIVERSE CONTEXTS

Although content throughout the text has application across diverse settings, some special considerations and examples are worth reviewing. This section includes discussion of online programs incorporating clinical practica, as well as programs and opportunities for staff development with technologies.

Clinical Practicum Courses and Technologies

Some of the most common online programs, including RN to BSN and graduate nursing education programs, incorporate clinical practica. Consistent with the call for advancing nursing education (IOM, 2015). these programs continue to grow. Many of these programs are completely or almost entirely online, presenting challenges as to how to best incorporate clinical practicum components. With large increases in these programs, it is important to identify ways that technology can help advance program quality.

For example, advanced clinical courses in graduate nursing and RN to BSN programs are common but have unique differences from traditional programs. These programs are often online and have students work with preceptors. The triangle of faculty, preceptor, and student requires enhanced ways to use technology to learn together and document progress. Preceptors play an important role when working with practice students at a distance. Technology becomes especially important in these practica, for example, in directing attention to how one communicates with and orients distance students and preceptors. This includes, for example, feedback and clinical evaluation components. E-Learning management systems and web-based resources such as online document management systems provide opportunities to orient all team members to course structure and process. Documenting distance clinical activities via electronic logs and e-portfolios are additional examples.

What if you are leading a practicum course? How can technology help students orient, engage, and move successfully through the courses? Key points to consider in online courses with practica include the following.

- **Preceptor:** Partnering with a preceptor and faculty team, students develop contracts outlining specific course goals and approaches. This provides a mutual guide for all to understand work to be completed and evaluative components to be addressed.

- **Contract:** Your students will be working with diverse populations and contexts, making the practicum similar to an independent study. As in an independent study, the contract is an important document, showing how course objectives will be met. Students meet with preceptors to identify the best approaches for completing contracts and try to meet needs of the clinical agency as well. Particularly at the graduate level, it is important to name the products that will help document course activities.
- **Clinical logs:** Clinical logs provide a type of student tracking system. Although early tracking systems were handwritten logs, the use of electronic tracking systems such as Typhon help students not only track their clinical hours, but also use data entered to help name their populations (practicum course and Typhon examples are further discussed in Chapter 13).
- **e-Portfolios:** e-Portfolios provide another opportunity for documenting clinical practica accomplishments. The use of an e-portfolio to document progress, especially for courses at a distance, can provide a valuable summary of contracted work, practicum products, and student reflective comments about the experience can be key components.
- **Reflection:** Portfolios without reflective summaries might be considered just a stack of documents. The benefits of student reflection include clearly naming and describing products developed, the reasons that they are important, and the ways that best practices have been incorporated.

Staff Development and Interprofessional Education

Technologies can help in interprofessional education (IPE) and staff development, including use of media such as individual webinars/podcasts and online programs. Common staff development challenges including rapid deployment of content and rapid healthcare system changes, call for educational best practices in staff development. As clinical practice with technology advances, education needs also change. Education for staff needs to be an efficient process and not take valuable time away from patient care. Although online education provides a unique opportunity to meet the needs of nursing staff with varied schedules and in varied settings, there can be challenges for new educators.

Podcasts/webinars and online programs: Recalling the best teaching and learning practices you have been reading about, do a quick self-assess of a recent webinar you have presented or participated in as a student. Was content engaging? Was active learning evident? How was learning and application evaluated? What were outcomes?

Similar principles for classroom and online teaching apply across educational venues. Staff need easily accessible, effective online education. Podcasts/webinars are easily accessible resources and provide learning versatility at almost any time or place. These can be important tools in maintaining ongoing quality improvement (QI) in education for patients and staff (as well as mentoring students). Similar to the best practices with more traditional class rooms, these teaching and learning modes are best when designed to keep students engaged. This includes approaches that engage staff not only for listening to the information, but also activities that focus on applying the information in clinical care.

Educational Partnerships: Schools and clinical agencies can focus more on partnering to improve student learning and readiness for practice. Opportunities for sharing/working together with both academia and IPE partners exist. This is another opportunity in which the Internet addresses previous IPE challenge of being in the same room at the same time. They are relevant, for example, to broad audiences for team-based clinical updates and sharing of new teaching and learning strategies. These approaches can provide partnering opportunities with IPE, sharing expertise with speakers from diverse specialties and professions, as well as providing opportunity for IPE discussions.

Another example for preparing clinical partners to work together involves combining clinical agencies and academia in the online classroom. As noted, diverse semester schedules, diverse settings, and other challenges have been noted as problems for bringing diverse professions together. An example of an IPE online program for health profession educators is provided in Exhibit 16.2. After reviewing this example, think about your current programs doing something similar. How many ways would your school and clinical agencies partner with technologies? Are there other needs/opportunities for which you could advocate?

Staff Development and Systems Approaches

Faculty and clinical staff onboarding: Onboarding is a common issue whether in academia or a clinical agency. Starting a new position can be a confusing time. A common challenge for both academic and clinical agencies, orienting new staff and faculty can present challenges that, if not handled well, can impact staff/faculty retention and patient care. Orientations to key technologies, such as electronic health record systems (EHRS) will be a part of this. There is value in online education that provides enduring resources for staff.

Must-know information for all units includes locating where resources are and knowing how things are done including policy and procedure protocols. Typically, this requires not only knowing the clinical education requirements for employment, such as safety and infection control, but also learning the clinical EHRS. Onboarding/orientation can be enhanced with web repositories to help. Ready access to resources in a well-organized system online helps initially and when follow-up is needed. Considering how best to present this information initially involves considering the best teaching and learning practices.

EXHIBIT 16.2

INITIATING IPE PARTNERSHIPS IN ACADEMIA—ONE SCHOOL'S EXAMPLE

Our current experiences relevant to interprofessional education and teamwork relate to the development of an on ongoing health professions educator certificate program. Leadership experiences with this program have been positive. During most semesters, we have a variety of disciplines (physical therapy, occupational therapy, dietetics, speech therapy) in our educator courses, along with our graduate nursing graduates. An overview and noted value of this program is summarized in a recent article.

For health professionals, learning together can be a strategy that facilitates working together. Student diversity provides both a challenge and the strength of the certificate program. Online IPE provides a unique opportunity to bring together different healthcare professions (avoiding the need for rigorous attention to varying semester and clinical location schedules among the disciplines). As students share their projects with each other at online discussions, they also share what makes each profession similar and different as they discuss common and unique teaching issues; all gain from the diverse experiences as they question and critique each other. The flexible, broad conceptual approach of course modules allows diverse students opportunity to package the learning activities and courses to meet unique needs (Bonnel & Tarnow, 2015).

IPE, interprofessional education.

As with academia, both new staff and the organization benefit when the best teaching and learning practices are used to help orient. Combined with a mentor, this can be a good start. Whether initial presentations are a classroom- or a webinar-type approach, the best teaching and learning practices are called for to make the best use of time. Questions for the staff educator to consider include the following: Which technology and teaching practices work best for a given situation? Can the Internet, learning management systems, or other in-house systems be useful? Also, simulations, as discussed earlier, provide good competency check-off opportunities. To this mix, remember to add a mentor or coach to provide ongoing support and guidance.

As you review your academic agency practices for onboarding new faculty, what similarities and differences do you find for onboarding at clinical agencies? What ways can technology help with ongoing support and mentoring for these individuals? Are there further opportunities for online discussion boards and e-communications? If you were creating an online handbook that connected to online resources to orient new staff or new faculty, what would be in your table of contents?

Evaluation from a system perspective: What is our QI for the specific programs we teach? How do we identify the impact of our continuing education (CE) programs? Evaluating staff education outcomes incorporates evaluation principles for students or patient evaluation, as discussed earlier.

A systems focus reminds us that this education is all about the outcomes. Competent staff are best situated to provide good patient outcomes. We are seeking ways to evaluate the performance of staff after a CE offering to see if change has taken place. This information is then incorporated into our program reports.

Staff development requires that education outcomes are documented in terms of staff satisfaction, knowledge, and behavior improvements. Technology can also help document staff development and outcomes from a unit/systems perspective. Asking questions such as the following can be helpful: Was this program or intervention effective? Who among the program's participants benefited most? What might be the reasons for the program's successes and failures?

Packaging these educational outcomes incorporates not only the individual, but also the applications of systems perspectives and QI. Showing improved staff behaviors (and patient care) is primarily why staff development exists, so it is important to document outcomes that staff are gaining. Although showing program attendance numbers and satisfaction ratings can be a part of this, it helps to think beyond this to system outcomes. Benefits to the systems approach include relating patient and unit outcomes and improvements to education and providing data for further QI needs and decision making. Examples are as follows:

- Use data to monitor care process outcomes (patient care) and use technology to organize and document system-wide outcomes, going beyond the individual patient level to the care system level. Staff development can help convey the importance of this to staff and share selected tools to help with this systems-type project (i.e., following patients from admit to discharge, their status, progress, and outcomes).
- For example, in a rehabilitation unit, nursing staff are concerned about documenting improving/positive outcomes for patients who have strokes. In a systems model, an evidence-based assessment tool is used to monitor patient outcomes. Sample tools on a rehabilitation unit, for example, could include nationally recognized tools, such as the Functional Independence Measure and the National Institutes of Health Stroke Scale. These tools can serve as a common language in helping to assess patients and document their progress on improvement goals. As patient outcomes are monitored over designated times, it provides staff feedback.
- In addition, as a part of this system, data can be used to help document staff development. All nursing staff have to demonstrate competency in using these tools and document yearly certification in using them.
- Other units can be asked to consider how technologies can help implement and document unit system outcomes, showing good, safe, patient care and staff competency. This can help promote evidence-based care for enhanced outcomes as well as its documentation.

Technology and staff development in the rural setting: The broad expectations of staff development in rural settings, as well as the benefits of technology, are conveyed by Rhonda Klaus (Exhibit 16.3). Describing the opportunities that technology provides in her rural setting, she emphasizes the import of understanding teaching and learning best practices and how

EXHIBIT 16.3

TEACHING WITH TECHNOLOGIES—RURAL STAFF DEVELOPMENT TIPS FROM CHAMPIONS

Rhonda D. Klaus, MSN, RN

1. *What is your current position like, relevant to using technology to engage individuals and teams in staff development?* My current position encompasses multiple technologies to engage individuals and teams in staff development. Examples include email, webinars, simulation laboratories, PowerPoint presentations, conference calls, internet TV, and smartphones. These modalities allow me to reach various audiences more conveniently. In many instances, the technology allows for a more realistic or real-time dissemination of the information, therefore reducing or eliminating information delays.

2. *What formal or informal education or training have you had in your current position?* Formal education for my current position consists of periodic scheduled meetings with the information technology (IT) department and product vendors regarding the use of their technology. The facility with which I am affiliated also requires completion of particular e-learning on hire and annually. Informal education received is composed of on-the-job training on an as-needed basis.

3. *Why is engagement for teaching and learning in staff development important to understand?* Engagement for teaching and learning in staff development is important to understand because it is the foundation on which we grow and sustain future educators and staff. To fail at engaging staff is to fail the facility as a whole. When staff are engaged, it enhances motivation for more purposeful action, and staff tend to be more invested in the success of their colleagues and the facility.

4. *What ways do you see staff benefiting from a better understanding of technology use, both as individuals and in teams?* Technology is constantly evolving, providing multiple benefits for nurse educators involved with staff development. Having a good working knowledge of technology resources allows individuals to collect and manage data, network with other individuals/organizations, and conveniently provide education to various audiences. Understanding technology allows teams to function more cohesively, provides immediate access to other team members/departments, and provides an important avenue for managing quality patient care.

5. *What are key points that nurse educator students would need to understand related to technology and teaching and learning issues in staff development?* Key points regarding technology use for nurse educator students include assessing your audience and considering how best to present educational content. For example, how adept is your audience with technology? Do they have access to technology resources, and are they compliant with your system? In addition, not all educational content may lend itself to being taught effectively with technology. Other key points are being knowledgeable about your technology system and remaining current with updates. It is important to know your IT contacts in case you experience issues with the function of the technology, along with monitoring its effectiveness. Are the recipients of the education in the technology format chosen receiving and understanding the information delivered?

6. *How do you manage to keep staff focused on learning?* When providing education, it is important to try to incorporate various learning styles (visual, auditory, interactive) to facilitate a positive and successful educational experience for students. In addition to audio/visual technology, interactive activities such as games or simulations are often good at keeping the audience interested. Many of these activities use technologies to facilitate active learning.

(continued)

7. **What are select challenges and facilitators for incorporating the use of technology to engage individuals on select topics in staff development? Challenges:** Select challenges include the readiness of colleagues and students to use technology. Some individuals may not feel prepared or may simply be resistant to change. Budget constraints remain a challenge because technology needs to be supported and updated on a routine basis. Finding time to implement professional development for those delivering the education is another challenge. At times, receiving necessary support from administration may be challenging. **Facilitators:** Select facilitators include the ability to reach a wide audience at various times (because of time/scheduling constraints) with technology. Another facilitator is the need for just-in-time education. Technology allows for rapid delivery of time-sensitive information to the necessary recipients. Technology allows immense creativity in the development of the education to be delivered. It allows the minutest details to be explained or demonstrated in a manner that is more easily understood by most learners.

8. **What tips would you like to share with new or future nurse educators about teaching with technology in staff development?** Advice for new or future nurse educators about teaching with technology includes being proactive with your own education opportunities. A prepared educator is more likely to be able to meet the challenges and needs of the target audience. Do not be afraid to experiment with various technologies and learning styles. Some methods may work better for some individuals/groups than others. The more diverse the tool kit, the more likely you will be successful in engaging a variety of learners.

technology allows her to reach multiple audiences at multiple times. Another example she relates is how when units do not have resources for journals and medical library subscriptions, the Internet (and guidance in how to find the best practices) serves as an excellent resource.

Partnerships, Healthcare Agencies, and Academia

Interprofessional and collaborative partnerships are considered key concepts to the future of nursing education. Nursing programs and affiliated health systems are missing benefits of enhanced collaboration and innovation if they are not working together. Examples include optimizing resources and learning together for future workforce development (Manatt Health Project Team, 2016). The following examples include academic and clinical partnering for QI, including graduate student projects and sharing of teaching and learning opportunities and resources such as EHRS.

Sharing QI: One opportunity includes academia working with clinical agencies to incorporate the concepts of QI for knowledge sharing such as Doctor of Nursing Practice (DNP) projects. A goal is for students to graduate with skills and expectations to start practice QI projects. As future clinical leaders, there is value in learning to work collaboratively at the student level. Technology can be used to help develop and maintain projects with clinical partnering opportunities for graduate and undergraduate students. Student assignments might incorporate a clinical partnership opportunity like the following QI projects. Each of these projects was completed in partnership with clinical agencies using technologies, including chart audits with EHRS and electronic surveys. Consistent with QI approaches, results were shared with each agency for further agency QI work. Final projects were shared at DNP public meetings, including live-streaming via web-conferencing software. Examples that address agency processes in comparing standards of care and providing ideas for additional student projects include the following:

- In partnering with a primary care clinic: Chronic Kidney Disease Awareness and Prevention of Progression (Coffin, 2017)
- In partnering with a mental health services agency: Improving Diabetes Care Delivery in an Integrated Health Clinic (Robinson, 2017)
- In partnering with a large hospital: Evaluation of Unit Based Councils (Curtis, 2016)

Sharing technology resources: As discussed throughout, technologies such as EHRS and high-fidelity simulation are important as learning tools and for learning across diverse settings, including classroom, online, laboratories, and clinical. Both academia and clinical agencies want positive student outcomes, so how can all help? Examples include the following:

- Gain further technology resources for EHRS or a high-fidelity simulations center. Particularly when student access is an issue, sharing resources such as technologies is an example. Just as a proposal was considered for documenting need and approaches for new courses, a proposal can also be a useful tool for gaining and sharing needed resources.
- Help faculty learn to write a proposal for needed technologies. This can include one-on-one mentoring as well as providing resources such as proposal templates.

SUMMARY

Strategic planning with a people focus and collaborative teamwork is needed when considering new technologies. In your faculty role, you will be taking major roles in mentoring faculty colleagues to new technologies. As you learn about new technologies and informatics concepts, it will be important for you to engage faculty in discussions regarding the value of adding these concepts or strategies to your curriculum. You will also have leadership and mentoring roles with clinical partners and teams.

ENDING REFLECTIONS FOR YOUR LEARNING NOTEBOOK

1. What is the most important content that you learned in this chapter?
2. What are your plans for using the information provided in this chapter in your future teaching endeavors?
3. What are your further learning goals?

GUIDELINES FOR TEACHING AND LEARNING WITH TECHNOLOGIES

Quick Teaching Tips

1. Help students use reflective assignments to identify strengths and weaknesses from their mentoring approaches.
2. Help students engage in curriculum discussions that relate to new content needs such as NI.
3. Engage students in compare-and-contrast discussions or assignments to identify similarities (and differences) in traditional academia and staff development.
4. Engage students in discussions or assignments, to address benefits in partnering with academia and clinical agencies to share clinical talent and resources.

Questions for Further Reflection

Review and select from the following questions for colleague discussions (or reflective notebooks).

1. What is your initial definition of a mentor?
2. What current ways are you engaged in mentoring?
3. What formal or informal approaches are you using?
4. Share with us a mentoring situation you were engaged in: What worked? What did not? What are you learning from our resources that might have helped improve this situation?
5. What makes mentoring different (or similar) for the following:
   - MS, DNP, or PhD faculty?
   - Different faculty generations?
   - Part-time or full-time faculty; full faculty role or clinical faculty only?

LEARNING ACTIVITIES

The purpose of this learning activity is to reflect on technologies and informatics concepts and processes within your curriculum. Choose from one of the following activities.

Curriculum assignment: After reviewing the appropriate AACN essentials related to NI for your course level, consider the following questions.

- Where is NI in your curriculum? (It may work the best to review course objectives if there is not a separate informatics course). Are you happy with your findings?
- What is the leader's role in informatics integration in your program?
- What additional leadership issues like IPE teams and consortiums that could be considered?

Meeting participation: Ask students to observe a planning or curriculum meeting to better learn the processes of curriculum decisions in their agency. Observations can be guided by reflective questions such as: What are the processes for putting a course/program together about NI and placing it in the context of your broader educational program? What can you learn from participating in a curriculum meeting or interview a committee member? Who are the people involved in this endeavor? What is the process for getting things done in your organization? What surprises you that you learn from this activity?

ONLINE RESOURCES FOR FURTHER LEARNING

This resource review can help you gain ideas and resources for ongoing and future work. The following websites have particular reference in guiding ongoing development practices in champions roles with informatics and technologies.

- QSEN Institute. This resource provides diverse learning activities for helping meet QSEN competencies. qsen.org/competencies
- The National Organization of Nurse Practitioner Faculties (NONPF). This organization is focused on graduate education for nurse practitioners. www.nonpf.org
- AACN Essentials: These documents focus on essential competencies for nursing graduates from baccalaureate through graduate education. www.aacnnursing.org/Education-Resources/AACN-Essentials
- The Association for Nursing Professional Development (ANPD). This organization works to advance the specialty practice for staff to ultimately enhance patient outcomes. www.anpd.org

REFERENCES

Bonnel, W., & Tarnow, K. (2015). Preparing health professions' educators via online certificate program: Structure and strategies for quality. *Nurse Educator*, 40(1), 51–54. doi:10.1097/NNE.0000000000000100

Coffin, M. (2017). *Chronic kidney disease awareness and prevention of progression.* University of Kansas DNP Project.

Curtis, S. (2016). *Evaluation of unit based councils.* University of Kansas DNP Project.

Institute of Medicine. (2015). *Assessing progress on the IOM report the future of nursing.* Washington, DC: National Academies Press.

Larson, L. R. (2017). *Perceptions and experiences of baccalaureate nursing program leaders related to nursing informatics* (Doctoral dissertation). University of Kansas Medical Center, Kansas City, KS.

Manatt Health Project Team. (2016). *Advancing healthcare transformation: A new era for academic nursing.* American Association of Colleges of Nursing. Retrieved from http://www.aacnnursing.org/Portals/42/Publications/AACN-New-Era-Report.pdf

National League for Nursing. (2006). The mentoring of nurse faculty tool kit. Retrieved from http://www.nln.org/professional-development-programs/teaching-resources/toolkits/mentoring-of-nurse-faculty

Phillips, S. L., & Denison, S. T. (2015). New faculty tips on having a successful mentoring experience. Retrieved from https://tomprof.stanford.edu/posting/1564

Robinson, J. (2017). *Improving diabetes care delivery in an integrated health clinic.* University of Kansas DNP Project.

Zachary, L. J. (2000). *The mentor's guide: Facilitating effective learning relationships.* San Francisco, CA: Jossey-Bass. Retrieved from http://media.wiley.com/product_data/excerpt/2X/04709077/047090772X-259.pdf

CHAPTER 17

Into the Future: Nurse Educators, Teaching Technologies, and Self-Directed Lifelong Learning

CHAPTER GOAL

Be reflective educators and look toward the future with a lifelong learning frame.

BEGINNING REFLECTION

1. What are your thoughts about future pedagogies and technology and student education?
2. What learning goals for your teaching-with-technologies work will you build on to stay current?
3. What models guide your scholarly work and planning for further technology projects?

Overheard: *What if?*

We are being asked to teach in ways we have not been taught and with tools we have not used. We are experiencing changing roles as faculty when we add technologies to our teaching. We negotiate new roles, sometimes dealing with internal conflict as we move from using more traditional teaching methods to integrating technologies that may not even have been invented when we attended our initial nursing programs. The learning curve is large and calls for our best self-directed learning skills. The call for new skills for a new age is described by Porter-O'Grady and Malloch (2014). We negotiate new roles as we consider what technologies can be used to enhance student learning.

Change as a Certainty

As noted throughout the text, change is the one certainty in the future of education. We do not know what the future holds in technology, but we can hypothesize that rapid, ongoing change will occur. When the authors started teaching, for example, the Internet had never been used in education. Preparing to teach students' new technologies and to teach using new technologies requires accepting that technology will change and that we will need to stay flexible. Educational technology, information management, and clinical practice technology are three frames to guide our future technology work (Skiba, Connors, & Jeffries, 2008). Identifying broad concepts and models within each of these frames helps us maintain a pedagogical base that moves us forward.

The uniqueness of patients and clinical settings calls for creative approaches to use and further test evidence-based practices. This is especially important in a rapidly changing healthcare environment. The goal is to gain faculty and students who are confident in using technologies to develop creative approaches in new, changing systems of care. Faculty then need to be creative in helping students gain traditional competencies in unique care settings. The future of nursing report, in synthesis of needs and evidence in the nursing profession, supports helping students seek strategies beyond the traditional solutions (Institute of Medicine [IOM] 2011, 2015).

Even as we gain a tool set for teaching with technologies, technology will continue to change, with many newer means emerging to promote student learning. The teacher as learner gains a synthesis of key points from this text as the basis for further projects, recalling that traditional pedagogies and emerging educational best practices help guide our work. This book has provided a collage of skills and thoughts for taking us into our changing classroom and clinical settings. Reflecting on the concepts in this book assists in planning the use of technology in our classrooms. This chapter reminds us to be reflective educators, to collaborate in future learning practices, and to look toward the future with a lifelong learning frame.

BEING A REFLECTIVE EDUCATOR

A reflective educator looks back and considers what has or has not been accomplished. A reflective educator is one who makes teaching and learning visible or clearly communicates the work of educators to others. Bernstein, Burnett, Goodburn, and Savory (2006) reflect on the importance of documenting what we do as teachers to help our learners achieve. As faculty, we can name what we do, considering what has worked well and what needs further work in our teaching and learning projects.

Readers are reminded about self-directed learning and lifelong learning concepts. We cannot prepare students well for the future unless we incorporate into our teaching the current technologies they will need to function in their profession and in the future. Our text has provided a toolkit of approaches for teaching technologies and teaching our students about technologies.

Teaching by the Evidence

MODELS TO GUIDE

The Integrated Learning Triangle for Teaching With Technologies (Exhibit 1.3), introduced in this text, has the advantages of showing quick reminders of key pieces that need to fit into teaching with technology considerations and lesson planning. As suggested in this model, opportunities exist for building on current best educational practices, as well as contributing to these best practices.

EVIDENCE-BASED TEACHING

Although healthcare professionals want best evidence for clinical practice, faculty also need an evidence base for their pedagogy or teaching practice. Best teaching requires us to give thoughtful attention to the ways that we structure our teaching and learning methods to ensure that we are basing our practices on the best evidence. Specific teaching concepts, such as concept mapping or problem-based learning, can be reviewed to identify the evidence base. Oermann (2009) notes the need for research to further develop the body of literature for health profession educators and suggests some beginning approaches.

Contributing to the Evidence and Sharing Our Successes

Although teaching by the evidence has been emphasized throughout the text, we also need to focus on our own educational scholarship and opportunities to contribute to best teaching practices and the generation of further educational research questions. The National League for Nursing (NLN, 2003) nurse educator competencies include sharing through scholarship as a major competency. Competency 7 of this document highlights engaging in scholarship, including the following themes: have an evidence base for teaching and learning, have a spirit of inquiry, engage in designing and implementing scholarly activities, disseminate teaching scholarship, develop proposals for varied initiatives, and demonstrate qualities of a scholar. We have as much responsibility to share our successful teaching strategies as we do our research studies. With the rapid pace of change, there is a particular need for sharing evaluative projects at this time.

Boyer's scholarship model. Boyer's (1990) classic framework provides direction in documenting our educational scholarship. Known as the scholarship of teaching and learning (SOTL), Boyer's work acknowledges faculty educational scholarship, as well as faculty clinical research, supporting that scholarship is not limited to clinical discovery research. His framework is based on teaching, application, integration, and discovery. Key points to recall are that being a scholar requires being prepared to find scholarship in diverse situations, working on something you are passionate about, and turning a project into an evaluative study by making sure it uses a systematic approach and is well packaged via a proposal that includes good evaluative measures. Once the project is completed and peer reviewed, plans for presenting and publishing are indicated. Specific to teaching and application scholarship, for example, faculty might develop an online learning object or activity, implement and evaluate it, and then share it so that others can learn from it. As indicated, this process includes naming and packaging the object or activity, having it peer reviewed, and then publishing it (Huber & Hutchings, 2005). Technology teaching and learning repositories and online educational journals make it easier than ever to share our products with diverse audiences.

Technology and the SOTL. The increased use of technology has pushed us to examine how we teach. This scholarship approach also engages us as reflective educators and provides a form of continuous quality improvement as we reflect on what we have done and then strive to continuously make our teaching better. Opportunities for teaching with technology provide an excellent time to examine the quality of our teaching work. Creating one's own quality improvement is as basic as reflecting on process and outcomes in our courses. We can use tools such as satisfaction surveys that are already in place. Questions are tools to keep us thinking and moving forward in our quality improvement. Generating good questions is a part of effective reflective practice, helping us guide our planning (what is working), as well as to consider opportunities for further study. Particularly with our rapidly changing technological world, questions provide guidance in the many areas that will continue to evolve.

Benefits to the Scholarship of Teaching and Learning

SOTL supports a spirit of inquiry to guide us into the future. Technology projects serve as excellent exemplars for scholarly projects. Presenting and publishing our work help others learn from our challenges and gain from our successes in projects specific to teaching with technologies. This provides a way to pass on what we have learned about teaching and educational best practices. If we are not sharing our own learning, it can be lost (see Exhibit 17.1). Faculty can guide students in educational scholarship using strategies such as the following:

- Synthesizing the literature on topics unique to concepts related to teaching and learning with technologies and developing strategies/protocols for underdeveloped topic areas
- Guiding quality improvement projects that address the use of best practices, attention to the needs of diverse students, and opportunities for practice improvements
- Guiding in packaging products in meaningful ways that can benefit faculty colleagues, students, and ultimately patients
- Disseminating scholarly products that are systematically documented, synthesized, and situated in the context of the professional literature

---

EXHIBIT 17.1

BENEFITS TO SOTL PROJECTS

- The scholarship of teaching and learning provides rich representation/description of our educational projects.
- Evaluation/evidence can lead to the generation of new project questions and questions for further educational research.
- The benefits of being reflective educational practitioners are evident and include opportunities for self-assessment and ongoing quality improvement in our teaching.
- Faculty gain opportunities to share and learn from one another's projects; the sharing can help create a learning community in our programs.
- Faculty gain the opportunity to organize/document our teaching protocols and to name what it is we do.
- The scholarship of teaching and learning demonstrates our thoughtful attention to our teaching and our efforts to continue to improve our practices within our changing nursing student populations and programs.

SOTL, scholarship of teaching and learning.

TOOLS FOR SCHOLARSHIP

E-Portfolios as Tools for Beginning Scholarship

Preparing students for advancing practice and future scholarship is part of life-long learning. It involves showing or documenting that learning is occurring, whether documenting basic competency or learning a new specialty. Portfolios provide a useful strategy for documenting either basic learning or specialty learning. As new graduates' focus extends beyond basic, general practice information, portfolios can support their ongoing learning and its documentation. Not all specialties are well developed, so e-portfolios can be particularly useful in guiding students in specialty development.

E-portfolios, or more generic professional portfolios, provide a way of describing and documenting student skills and accomplishments. Specifically, a portfolio characterizes one's expertise by highlighting strengths as projects are completed and documented. In addition to providing evidence of one's work, portfolios provide an opportunity for self-analysis and reflection. Although portfolios have existed for many years in hard-copy format, the ability to complete them via electronic systems or even personal word-processing programs provides enhanced opportunities for updating and sharing.

Diverse E-Portfolio Approaches

As students prepare for careers, there is value in using portfolios to help document their accomplishments. Examples of portfolios with varying purposes, helpful in future careers, include the following:

- Career portfolios—a faculty career-focused portfolio that documents a range of aspects specific to our practice, education, research, and leadership

- Project portfolios—a faculty portfolio developed around one specific project showcasing both process and accomplishments
- Student learning portfolios—a student-generated portfolio that documents specified aspects of student learning

Reflection and E-portfolios

Portfolios are valuable, not just for packaging completed assignments, but for engagement of students to reflect and self-assess about their accomplishments. Reflections can help engage students in their responsibility for learning and sharing important products with others. Design prompts and questions to guide reflections include the following: What skills have you improved on and gained confidence in? What has been surprising? What has been important to your practice? What sets the stage for goal setting as to what next?

TEACHING SCHOLARSHIP, TECHNOLOGY, AND INTERPROFESSIONAL CLINICAL PARTNERS

Teaching with technology is not a solitary endeavor in healthcare. Working and learning collaboratively with interprofessional colleagues and clinical partners benefits students' learning for future practice. The IOM (2003) recommends using technology and working as interprofessional teams to further clinical learning goals. Interprofessional education involves two or more academic disciplines. Learning as teams can help students gain beginning insights into various team members' perceptions of their role in practice. In the same way, faculty can partner to learn from what other disciplines are doing in technology-related pedagogies.

Partnering with other healthcare professions for traditional interprofessional classroom education is a strategy that some have found challenging. Diverse campus settings, diverse semester and clinical schedules, and increased faculty responsibilities are sample challenges. Problems can exist (e.g., finding common settings and times to hold interprofessional classes). An option that avoids the time and space (i.e., classroom) challenges involves partnering to develop and deliver interprofessional continuing education via the Internet. Online asynchronous technology is especially useful at a time when schedules can make it difficult to get students from different disciplines together.

In addition, high-fidelity simulation technology has become increasingly popular in providing important opportunities for interprofessional education. Opportunities with simulators include learning improved communication modes and gaining insight into the perspectives of other disciplines. These learning opportunities also provide a broader systems approach to learning that avoids compartmentalization of basic science, behavioral science, and clinical disciplines as recommended by the Quality and Safety Education for Nurses Institute (QSEN; 2017) and the IOM (2003). These resources also note that further development of what works in clinical education is needed, including

EXHIBIT 17.2

SHARING INTERPROFESSIONAL RESOURCES

Sample learning opportunities for working as part of interprofessional teams include the following:

- *Classroom and online learning opportunities.* One way to promote interprofessional education includes extending collaborative learning efforts via technology. Informatics concepts and courses are well suited to interprofessional education. Working as teams and using informatics are two of the recommended competencies from the IOM (2003) and the QSEN Institute (2017).
- *Online sharing of interprofessional resources.* Sharing interprofessional resources for critique exposes nurses to new ways of approaching problems as we learn about tools of the various disciplines.
- *Safety projects and interprofessional learning.* Technology plays a central role in providing better communication and promoting a safer patient care environment. With the focus on safe, quality care, the entire healthcare team, including the patient as part of that team, is engaged. Our range for safety is broad, from teaching infant safety to helping older adults manage complex medication regimens. Our guiding assignment question might be, "How can students best learn to engage with patients, staff, students, and others in participating as members of the safety healthcare team?"

IOM, Institute of Medicine; QSEN, Quality and Safety Education for Nurses; SOTL, scholarship of teaching and learning.

the determination of what content matters most and what teaching strategies work best. Students' care for a variety of patients in a variety of settings can only be enhanced through better understanding of the roles of multiple disciplines. Exhibit 17.2 provides sample learning opportunities for working as part of interprofessional teams.

TEACHING WITH TECHNOLOGIES: INTO THE FUTURE

As both educators and learners, we need to stay motivated and continue to be self-directed learners if we are to keep up with this rapidly changing technology and the pace of clinical education. Varied learning approaches can be combined to help us keep up with ongoing and future changes. Future learning includes accessing just-in-time resources. For example, online tutorials or freely accessible online videos, as well as traditional written materials, are extensive. Just-in-time education is no longer simply nice to have but is often required on a regular basis. Sample suggestions for creating learning plans include the following:

- Gain web education, both formal and informal, including both pedagogical and clinical resources.
- Create informal learning plans based on trusted clinical organizational resources.

- Seek resources from national leadership in the clinical education arena, such as Technology Informatics Guiding Educational Reform (TIGER) the QSEN Institute.
- Seek out resources from professional nursing or interprofessional associations, such as the American Nurses Association or the American Geriatrics Society.
- Keep up an area of specialty interest via listservs and other electronic networks.
- Attend actual or virtual professional meetings.
- Scan program topics from online conference brochures.
- Participate in learning object repositories such as the Teaching, Learning, and Technology Group (www.tltgroup.org) and others.
- Continue formal coursework, such as courses on teaching with technologies (Bonnel, Wambach, & Connors, 2005).
- Mentor others by working with technology-invested younger faculty to blend seasoned educators' years of pedagogical experience with their enthusiasm for technology (or vice versa).
- Scan for current trends that influence and guide teaching with various technologies. A reflective educator scans the horizon and thinks about what is needed to stay current.
- Participate in national task forces. Opportunities that might previously have been cost-prohibitive (participation in state, national, and international organizations and their task groups) can now often be accomplished from the comfort of work or home offices.

CHANGING OUR EDUCATION TO FIT THE CHANGING WORLD

Looking back to the early IOM reports addressing healthcare quality and safety serves as a reminder of the important role educators have to play. These reports are key components in the current restructuring of healthcare; an important element of this restructuring is to eliminate gaps between education and practice. Healthcare provider education includes not only focusing on the reports' content, but also incorporating core competencies, including safety and quality care. This book has been about using technology to help us do this (see Exhibit 17.3 for a summary related to the IOM (2003) and health profession report).

Change is the one certainty in the future of education. What is cutting-edge today will quickly pass, replaced by newer technology. Technology has provided new ways to envision our teaching and learning approaches to help students gain needed competencies. As our younger, technology-savvy students move into clinical practice, they will be prepared to learn and build with technology resources. Examples of the ways in which students will use new technology include the following:

- Gaining experiences with mobile devices for keeping up with the evidence needed in their patients' care

EXHIBIT 17.3

QSEN INSTITUTE/IOM HEALTH PROFESSIONS EDUCATION REVISITED

The IOM (2003) provides faculty with direction in moving nursing education forward. *Technology* serves in uniting the IOM concepts, including the following examples:

- *Interprofessional practice*. Clinical team members are brought together in important ways to share data management via electronic health records and diverse technologies such as simulation laboratories and Internet-based programs.
- *Evidence-based practice*. Technology serves as a central tool in the search, access, critique, and synthesis of best evidence for practice. It helps move evidence to protocol formats that can be electronically shared, used, and evaluated.
- *Information management in quality improvement*. Informatics tools help in designing individual and population databases that serve the needs of patients, providers, and other healthcare system team members.
- *Client-centered care*. Care advances such as electronic information systems and the Internet help enhance patients as the center of the team, giving them access to data and resources for informed clinical decisions.

IOM, Institute of Medicine; QSEN, Quality and Safety Education for Nurses.

- Building opportunities for learning with the Internet and not just within the confines of an online course to gain evidence-based resources for the future
- Gaining confidence for their patient care responsibilities and future staff development roles in using high-tech simulators
- Learning skills in data management to promote the health of the populations for which they care

Preparing to teach with technologies in the future requires accepting that technology will change and that we will need to stay flexible. Selected take-home points from this chapter include the following:

- Use lifelong learning as more than a buzzword.
- Build bridges with interprofessional practice partners.
- Gain a mentor and community network of fellow learners.
- Identify strategies to scan the future and keep up.
- Evaluate what does and does not work in teaching with technologies for selected populations.
- Contribute to the scholarship of teaching, learning, and sharing best practices.

Sharing a teaching-with-technology project as scholarship, as previously noted, provides a way to continue learning and promotes quality in our teaching. Exhibit 17.4 provides ideas for a beginning write-up of a teaching project.

EXHIBIT 17.4

GUIDELINES FOR SHARING THE SCHOLARSHIP OF TECHNOLOGY PROJECTS

To share an assignment or a teaching project, use a project summary format that might be used in developing a professional portfolio or in beginning the steps for manuscript development. The descriptive sharing includes not only the assignment/project structure but also the challenges, strategies, process, and outcomes. For example, consider the following questions:

- What is the assignment/project?
- Why is it important?
- How is it designed (the structure, the process)?
- How do faculty and students participate or process roles?
- How are students evaluated? What are the outcomes?
- On completion, what was especially good or challenging about the project? What would you do differently next time?

SUMMARY

Basic teaching and learning principles can guide us in moving our teaching and learning with technologies into the future. Building on an evidence base and guiding our work with best practices and relevant theory can direct our teaching activities with new and emerging technologies. Technology challenges us to be innovative and creative as we help our students learn with and about educational technologies, clinical technologies, and informatics. In all cases, our goals continue to include developing professional, competent students prepared to enhance patient care.

ENDING REFLECTION FOR YOUR LEARNING NOTEBOOK

1. What is the most important content that you learned in this chapter?
2. What are your plans for using the information provided in this chapter in your future teaching endeavors?
3. What are your further learning goals?

GUIDELINES FOR TEACHING AND LEARNING WITH TECHNOLOGIES

Quick Teaching Tips

1. Consider roles and responsibilities in mentoring and being mentored.
2. Implement a portfolio project that showcases a teaching with technology assignment or class as a way to demonstrate educational scholarship.

3. Gain skills in peer review and project dissemination in sharing scholarship of teaching with technologies.

Further Questions for Reflection

As a reflective educator, consider the following reflective prompts to assist in further planning for teaching with technologies:

1. What strategies do we as educators need to consider in our teaching with technology plans to be a proactive rather than reactive part of the future?
2. What are your best successes in teaching with technologies? What is working best for you in teaching or learning with technology?
3. What strategies can help us make teaching scholarship more a part of our professional teaching careers or clinical educator roles?

Learning Activity: e-Portfolio

Your goal and the purpose of this assignment are to help advance the teaching and learning technologies specialty. Often, creating a project e-portfolio is a good start for sharing your SOTL with technologies. As faculty, ask yourself what teaching and learning project you are, or would like to be, implementing and evaluating. Brainstorm your current (or planned work) and generate a table of contents for the project or scholarly portfolio you want to develop.

Learning Activity: Mentoring and Scholarship Self-Assessment

The purpose of this assignment is to help your mentees self-assess on their scholarship needs. For example, using NLN Educators Competency 8, ask your mentee to assess and identify current learning needs for scholarship. This will incorporate clinical knowledge and experience for a proposed project, as well as teaching and learning with technologies knowledge and experience.

Online Resources for Further Learning

This resource review helps you gain ideas and resources for ongoing and future work. The following have particular reference in guiding ongoing teaching with technology projects:

- Tomorrow's Professor listserv. This ongoing listserv provides continued ideas for improving pedagogical skills. tomprof.stanford.edu/welcome
- "Emerging Perspectives on Learning, Teaching, and Technology." This online text, edited by Michael Orey, provides an example of an ongoing text-development process, as well as a text used for multiple purposes, and should provide reading into the future. textbookequity .org/Textbooks/Orey_Emergin_Perspectives_Learning.pdf

REFERENCES

Bernstein, D., Burnett, A., Goodburn, A., & Savory, P. (2006). *Making teaching and learning visible: Course portfolios and the peer review of teaching*. San Francisco, CA: Jossey-Bass.

Bonnel, W., Wambach, K., & Connors, H. (2005). A nurse educator teaching with technologies course: More than teaching on the web. *Journal of Professional Nursing, 21*(1), 59–65. doi:10.1016/j.profnurs.2004.11.002

Boyer, E. L. (1990). *Scholarship reconsidered: Priorities of the professoriate*. Princeton, NJ: Carnegie Foundation for the Advancement of Teaching.

Huber, M. T., & Hutchings, P. (2005). *The advancement of learning: Building the teaching commons*. San Francisco, CA: Jossey-Bass.

Institute of Medicine. (2003). *Health professions education: A bridge to quality*. Washington, DC: National Academies Press.

Institute of Medicine. (2011). *The future of nursing: Leading change, advancing health*. Washington, DC: National Academies Press.

Institute of Medicine. (2015). *Assessing progress on the IOM report the future of nursing*. Washington, DC: National Academies Press.

National League for Nursing. (2003). Core competencies of nurse educators. Retrieved from http://www.nln.org/professional-development-programs/competencies-for-nursing-education/nurse-educator-core-competency

Oermann, M. H. (2009). Evidence-based nursing education, leader to leader—National Council of State Boards of Nursing. Retrieved from https://www.ncsbn.org/Leader-to-Leader_Spring09.pdf

Porter-O'Grady, T., & Malloch, K. (2014). *Quantum leadership: A resource for healthcare innovation* (2nd ed.). Boston, MA: Jones & Bartlett.

Quality and Safety Education for Nurses Institute. (2017). QSEN competencies. Retrieved from http://qsen.org/competencies

Skiba, D. J., Connors, H. R., & Jeffries, P. R. (2008). Information technologies and the transformation of nursing education. *Nursing Outlook, 56*(5), 225–230. doi:10.1016/j.outlook.2008.06.012

Zachary, L. J. (2000). *The mentor's guide: Facilitating effective learning relationships*. San Francisco, CA: Jossey-Bass.

New Technology Readiness Inventory

The following inventory can help answer the why, how, and when of learning a new technology. Organized around the concepts of readiness, opportunity, and support, the inventory provides direction in identifying an individualized plan. Please reflect on the following items specific to a new technology with which you would like to teach.

1. For the *specific* technology, what is your:
   a. Readiness/motivation—What is your readiness to learn/gain comfort with the technology? Would you rate this as low, moderate, or high?
   b. Opportunity—What is available to you in terms of technology resources and environment? Are there opportunities to access the technology you hope to use?
   c. Support—Who is available (locally or at a distance) to mentor or coach you in teaching with a specific technology?
2. Based on your assessment, what learning goals will you set?
   a. Goal statement (includes your intention and time frame).
3. Based on your goals, what specific plan will you design to enhance your technology learning/comfort needs?
   a. Plan (includes two to three specific action steps).
4. What potential challenges exist or might limit your efforts? What strategies would be most likely to promote success?

Integrated Learning Triangle for Teaching With Technologies

The following guides flow from the Integrated Learning Triangle for Teaching With Technologies and can help answer the why, how, and when of using technology for a specific course, lesson, or assignment. Questions are organized around the mnemonic BEBOLDER to guide reflection. Consider the following items as you think about your plans for using technology:

- *Best teaching evidence and practices.* What evidence is available to guide implementation of a particular technology? What are recommended approaches?
- *Educational principles and theories.* What broad principles or theories, such as adult education theory, best fit student learning needs and teaching opportunities?
- *Beginning assessments.* What student learning needs are specific to the student level and content to be taught?
- *Objectives.* What is to be achieved in a specific course, lesson, or assignment? How can technology help?
- *Logistics/context.* What is the setting for teaching and learning? What physical resources are available? How many students are to be engaged? What are the strengths of available resource people to assist them?
- *Decision/fit.* What is the best technology fit for given learning needs and resources? What are the best teaching/learning activities to engage students?
- *Evaluation and feedback.* What is the evaluation plan? What feedback mechanisms are integrated into the course? How will you know if technology is helping students learn?
- *Review and revision.* How will you build quality improvement into your plan? What worked and what did not? What needs to be improved?

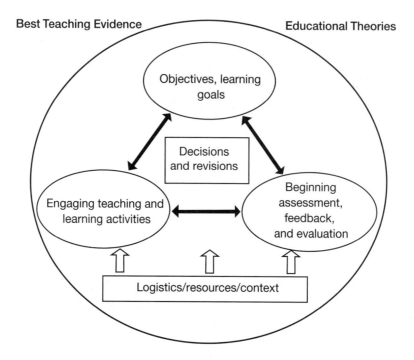

FURTHER QUESTIONS TO GUIDE REFLECTIONS

How does a particular technology best meet learning needs? For a particular course or assignment, will the technology:

- Help capture the concepts you are teaching?
- Assist students in meeting the objectives of the course?
- Help focus students' learning? Motivate students to become involved in learning?
- Help students make transitions to practice or focus on important concepts?

Also, for a given point in time:

- Is a particular technology worth the time and effort? (Would a less expensive technology work as well? What are the trade-offs?)
- What is the evidence for using the technology? (If there is limited evidence, is it consistent with good theory and educational principles?)
- Is the workload reasonable and well placed for both faculty and students?

Index

accomplishments, 96–97
ACES. *See* Advancing Care Excellence
　　for Seniors program
active auditory learning, 106–107, 154–155
adult education
　　concepts of, 17–18
　　pedagogies of, 215
　　theory of, 39, 104–105
adult learning theory, 31
Advancing Care Excellence for Seniors
　　(ACES) program, 213
aging population, 223
AHIMA. *See* American Health Information
　　Management Association
AHRQ. *See* Healthcare Research and
　　Quality
American Association for Higher Education,
　　48, 93, 117, 208
American Association of Colleges of
　　Nursing, 210, 226, 243
American Geriatrics Society, 262
American Health Information Management
　　Association (AHIMA), 19
American Nurses Association, 262
analysis, 125
andragogy, 4
applied learning, 105
　　assignments, 140
　　clinical teaching incorporating, 201
　　examples of, 143
　　reflection added to, 142
applied products, 141–142
applied technologies assignments, active
　　learning, 104–105
　　applied, 113, 140–141
　　assignments, 104–105, 109–110, 113
　　audio aspect of, 106–107
　　best practices related to, 105–106
　　learner engaged by, 50–51

PowerPoint and, 154–155, 162
　　visual aspect of, 107–108
approaches
　　to gaming, 174
　　to teaching, 105
　　variety of, 140
ARS. *See* automated response system
assessments, 118–119
　　of learning style, 23
　　of needs by faculty, 201
　　remediation and, 120–121
　　technology enhancing,120
assignments
　　active learning, 105–109, 109–110
　　allowing sharing, 96
　　authentic, 109–110, 141
　　of clinical learning lab, 201–202
　　design of, 202
　　engaging, 143
　　faculty developing, 64, 211
　　group, 93
　　meaningful, 110–111
　　observation, 110
　　online, 144
　　pocket, 216
　　preclass, 159
　　reflection as, 90, 111–112
　　repositories, 112
　　writing, 78–79
asynchronous learning, 134
audio
　　aspect of active learning, 106–109
　　casts, 160–161
　　examples of technology, 106–109
　　online students and, 8
　　strategies, 50
audiovisual learning, 109
authentic assignments, 110,
　　141–142

authentic learning, 105
automated response system (ARS), 117, 151.
    See also clickers
autonomy, 24, 34

Baby Boomers, 92
baseline
    data, 18
    for faculty, 133
BEBOLDER (Best Evidence, Educational
        theories, Beginning assessments,
        Objectives, Logistics, Decisions,
        Evaluation/Feedback, and
        Revisions), 9, 10, 13
beginnings, 94–95, 120
behavior, 98
behaviorists, 31
benchmarks, 18–19
best practice
    active learning related to, 105
    in clinical education, 215
    learning facilitated by, 140
    online teaching, 135
    pedagogies, 4
    strategies based on, 148
best teaching practices
    learning principles of, 35
    teaching principles of, 35
bias, 123
Boyer, Ernest, 257–258
Boyer's scholarship model, 257–258

Camtasia, 8, 11, 107, 160
Carnegie Mellon University, 5, 35,
        89, 92
CDC. *See* Centers for Disease Control
        and Prevention
CD-ROM, 108
Centers for Disease Control and
        Prevention (CDC), 190
Chickering, A. W., 5, 34–35, 106
class
    beginning of, 120
    closure of, 50
    discussion in, 79–80
    face-to-face, 21
    lesson plans for, 53
    nursing, 44–45
    orientation framing, 22
    pre/post, 49–50
    surveys, 95
classroom capture software, 160

classroom response systems.
        See Clickers
classrooms
    clickers in, 153–154
    EHR in, 192–193
    hardware in, 124
    moved to web, 4
    technology managed, 158–159
clickers, 124
    in classrooms, 152
clinical care, 207
clinical competencies, 126
clinical data management, 194
clinical education
    best practices in, 215
    changes in, 57
    pace of, 261
clinical evaluation, 208–209
clinical learning, 177–178
clinical learning lab, 200–201
    assignments of, 201–202
    purpose of, 202
clinical orientation, 52
clinical practice
    fundamental to nursing, 165
    IOM on, 39
    as part of nursing, 104
    technology, 6–7
clinical setting
    facilitation of, 205–206
    safety in, 215
    supervising, 205
    technology awareness
        in, 213
clinical teaching, 216
clinical tracking system, 208
clinical units, 204
closure, 50
coaching, 21–22
colleagues, 237, 252
communication tools, 82, 84
complexity theory, 32
computer-generated reminders, 82
concept mapping tools, 216
concepts, of adult education,
        17–18
constructivism, 31–32
content, 48–49
continuous quality improvement
        (CQI), 146–147, 189
course beginnings, 94–95, 120
CQI. *See* continuous quality
        improvement
critical care, 211

critical thinking
  in context, 188
  with EHR, 184–186
  enhancing, 207–208
  learning and, 75, 184
  teaching, 184
critique discussion, 62–63
cues
  nonverbal, 161
  verbal, 160
culture, 93
curricular issues, 191

data
  baseline, 187–188
  EHRS assignments, 188
  electronic systems, 188
  ethics to management of, 192
  implications of, 188
  learning about, 189
  management, 181, 195
  sets, 184, 194
databases, 61, 62
  online, 82
debate, about strategies 154
debriefing, 124, 169, 207
  of students, 208
design
  of assignments, 202
  of feedback, 149
  of online courses, 138–140
  of teaching, 18
digital citizenship, 98–99
digital images, 230
discussion
  in class, 79–80
  online, 142–144
  questions, 156
distance education, 160
  alternate classroom experience, 160–161
diversity
  campus, 260
  of culture, 93
  of learning community, 92
  multigenerational, 92
  of students, 7–8
  technology and, 93
DNP preceptor studio, 204
documentation, 207–208
documents
  repository of, 203
  reviews of, 142
DVDs, 108

EBP. See evidence-based practice
education
  distance, 160–161
  in games, 167
  healthcare, 199
  HFPS, 170
  nursing, 93
  online learning changing, 134–135
  patient, 143
  principles of, 50
  of the Web, 261
educational technology, 6
EHR. See electronic health records
e-learning. See online education
electronic gaming, 167
electronic health records (EHR),170–171,
    184, 189
  assessment form, 187–188
  assignments, 188
  for care planning, 188
  in classroom, 192–193
  critical thinking with, 184
  evolution of, 188
  as learning tool, 184–185
  Q & A, 185
electronic information systems, 188–189
electronic networks, 262
electronic repositories, 112
Elluminate-type programs/Camtasia, 160
email, 85
emotional learning, 89
endings, 96–98
enrichment, 25–26
e-portfolios
  career portfolios, 259
  project portfolios, 260
  student learning, 260
ethics
  of data management, 192
  guidelines to, 98
etiquette, 98–99
evaluation, 51–52, 118–119, 124–127
  feedback vs., 80
  formative vs. summative, 119
  module, 146
  norm vs. criterion-referenced, 119–120
  of peers, 123
  teaching related to, 118–121
evidence
  contribution to, 257–258
  teaching based on, 257
evidence-based practice (EBP),
    64–65, 113
experiential learning, 105

Facebook, 66, 80, 97, 100, 161
facilitation
    of clinical setting, 205
    of learning communities, 98–99
faculty
    assessment of needs by, 201
    assignments developed by, 64
    baseline for, 133
    changing roles for, 255–256
    classrooms needed by, 151
    clinical information conveyed by, 15–16
    clinical units orienting to, 204
    control of experiences, 126
    feedback sourced from, 121–122
    simulation orientation for, 174
faculty orientation to learning simulation, 173
feedback, 51–52, 80, 118–119, 124–127
    assessment activities, 176
    debriefing as, 123–124
    design of, 149
    evaluation vs., 80
    faculty as source of, 121–122
    forms of, 121–124
    immediate, 117
FIM. See Functional Independence
    Measure
fingertip technology, 60
Fink, L. D., 8–9, 17, 22–24, 38, 94, 134
Finkelman, A., 36–37
FIRE (focused program content, interactive
    teaching methods, reinforced
    learning, and evaluation), 51
flipped classroom, 158
format, 45
Functional Independence Measure
    (FIM), 193

gain web education, 261
games
    approach to, 175
    electronic, 167
gaming, 174
Gamson, Z. F., 5, 34–35, 106, 153
generation Xers, 92
geriatrics, 19
good communication techniques, 82
group introductions, 95

Healthcare Research and Quality (AHRQ)
    modules, 217
Health Information Technology Scholars
    Program (HITS), 207

Health Insurance Portability and
    Accountability Act (HIPAA), 192–206
health literacy, 59, 76, 84, 223
HFPS. See high-fidelity patient stimulation
high-fidelity patient simulation (HFPS),
    125–126, 169–171
    access to, 176
HIPAA. See Health Insurance Portability
    and Accountability Act
HITS. See Health Information Technology
    Scholars Program
humanistic learning theory, 31
hybrid learning
    active learning and PowerPoint, 154–155
    automated response systems, 153
    evidence-based review abstract, 154
    tools for interactive learning, 153–155
    web-based modules as a classroom
        adjunct, 155

idea structuring, 30–31
informatics, 181
    competency in, 3
    in health care, 182–183
    importance of, 182
    organizations supporting, 182–183
information
    accessing, 60–61
    model and theory, 35–36
    proliferation of, 151
    recommendations, 37
    reports, 36–37
    resources, 206
    technology, 189
    web changing, 57
information literacy, 5, 7, 17, 58–59
information management, 182–183
information systems, 183, 189
    importance of, 182–183
    teaching population and public
        health, 189
Institute of Medicine (IOM), 7, 29, 82, 199,
    220, 239
    on clinical expertise, 63
    core competencies of, 37
    on health care, 36
integrated learning triangle, 38, 45, 176–177
interactive television (ITV), 160
interdisciplinary clinical partners, 260–261
International Nursing Association for
    Clinical Simulation and Learning,
    167
interpretation of literature, 54, 122

interprofessional associations
American Geriatrics Society, 262
American Nurses Association, 81–82, 260–261
interprofessional education, 260
interview, 110, 142
IOM. *See* Institute of Medicine
ITV. *See* Interactive television

JCAHO. *See* The Joint Commission on the Accreditation of Healthcare Organizations
journals, 122

Kenner, C., 36, 82
kinesthetics, 51

learners
active learning engaging, 50–51
motivation of, 261
learning
etiquette of, 98–99
learning communities energizing, 91
principles of, 35
social spaces of, 80
storytelling improving, 110, 113
style, 23
time, 147–148
learning community
building of, 93–94
diversity of, 92
facilitator for, 95–96
learning energized by, 91
orienting, 95
learning management systems, 117, 124–125, 158–159
"Learning to Learn with Concept Mapping," 35, 38
lecture, 50
leadership
clinical practicum courses, 245–246
in diverse educational contexts, 245
partnerships, healthcare agencies, and academia, 251–252
podcasts/webinars, 246
staff development, 247–251
systems approaches, 247–249
technologies, 245–246
theories, 33

lesson plans
format of, 45
as organizing tools, 44
lifelong learning, 256
Long-Term Care Minimum Data Set (MDS), 188

management systems, 159
massive open online courses (MOOCs), 147
MDS. *See* Minimum Data Set
mentor, 241
middles, 95–96
millennials, 92
Minimum Data Set (MDS), 194
models and resources, 8–11
novice-to-expert, 60
traditional, 151
modules
AHRQ, 217
evaluation, 147
web-based, 155–158
monitoring, 183, 231
MOOCS. *See* massive online open courses
multipoint conferencing software, 160

National Database of Nursing Quality Indicators (NDNQI), 191
National League of Nursing (NLN), 168
National task forces, 262
NDNQI. *See* National Database of Nursing Quality Indicators
networks
community, 226
electronic, 262
informatics, 190
NLN. *See* National League of Nursing
nonverbal cues, 161
nursing informatics (NI), 191, 241

OASIS. *See* Outcome and Assessment Information
observation-type assignments, 142
online education, 133, 134
benefits of access and timeliness, 134
best practices, selected models, 135
continuous quality improvement, 146–148
of design in, 138–140
feedback, 144–145
online and self-directed learning, 134
practices in, 135–136

online learning, 133
online quizzes, 121
orientation
    class framed by, 22
    clinical, 54
    of learning community, 95
Outcome and Assessment Information
    Set (OASIS), 193

pacing, 145
patient education, 76, 143
patient portals, 223–224
pedagogy, 4–5, 181, 216
    of adult education, 215
    andragogy vs., 31
    behind online education, 135
    clinical learning lab and, 200–201
    flipped classroom, 158
    guidelines, 195
    importance of, 4
    teaching technology in partnership
        with, 9
PICO (Patient, Intervention, Comparison,
    Outcome), 65
Podcasts, 63, 76, 107, 113, 160
population health, 114–115, 224–227
PowerPoint, 148, 154–155
preclass assignments, 49, 159
purpose statement, 111

QSEN. See Quality and Safety Education
    for Nurses
Quality and Safety Education for Nurses
    (QSEN), 12, 19, 51, 74–75, 112,
    126, 176, 260
quality gap, 67
quality improvement, 20–21
quality matters rubric, 147, 150
questions, 172–173
    discussion, 156
    to students, 142

range of motion (ROM), 30, 178
reading literacy, 59
reflections, 260
reflective educator, 256–258
Reflective Reports assignment, 190
reflective self-assessments, 22–23
reflective writing, 122
remediation, 120–121
respiratory assessment study, 6
ROM. See range of motion

rubrics, 123, 168
    laboratory, 202–203
    Quality Matters program, 147

scholarship of teaching and learning
    (SOTL), 258–259
    benefits to, 258–259
    Boyer's scholarship model, 257–258
    e-portfolios as tool, 259–260
    guidelines for, 264
    interprofessional clinical partners,
        260–261
    teaching with technologies,
        261–262
SDL. See self-directed learning
self-assessment, 121–122
self-directed learning (SDL)
    based on learning assessments, 18
    identifying, 16–17
    lifelong learning linked to, 15, 16
    online learning and, 133
    theory background for, 17–18
set, 49
Shadow Health, 175
simulation-based education, 166–167
    evidence-based review abstract, 173
    facilitation and debriefing, 169
    high-fidelity patient simulation,
        169–171
    and objectives, 167–168
    orientation, 169
    outcomes, 167–168
    principles of, 167
    rubrics, 168
Simulation Innovation Resource Center
    (SIRC), 5, 168
SIRC. See Simulation Innovation
    Resource Center
Skype, 76
Snapchat, 66
social learning spaces, 80–81
social learning theory, 31
social spaces, online, 100
software, 124
    for Web conferencing, 160
SOTL. See scholarship of teaching and
    learning
standardized computer testing, 125
students
    graduate, 90
    public confidence in, 117
    reflection by, 121–122
    working together, 91

summarizing, 96
surveys, 95
systematic search, 61
synthesizing, 64
systems theory, 33, 191

teaching, 199
   approaches to, 209–210
   evaluation related to, 118–121
   information management, importance
      of, 182–183
teaching/learning activities, 176
technology
   advances in, 146
   assessment enhanced by, 120
   clinical evaluation, 208–209
   critical care and, 210–211
   developing course/program proposal,
      244–245
   diversity and, 93
   emerging, 126
   examples, 225–226
   faculty champions, 231–232
   and health literacy needs, 223–224
   leadership and mentoring roles
      with, 238
   mentoring tools, 238–239
   in patient education, 214–215, 221–222
   patient portals, 223
   patient safety and quality care, 209, 227
   phone nursing, 228
   point of care, 210–211
   population health, 226
   principles and useful mentoring tools,
      238–239
   safe, quality care, 227
   select, 124–127
   surgical care, 210–211
   systems, 82
   Telehealth, 228
   web-based education, 222–223
Technology Informatics Guiding Educational
   Reform (TIGER), 262

Telehealth, 228–231
The Joint Commission on the Accreditation
   of Healthcare Organizations
   (JCAHO), 193
TIGER. *See* technology Informatics Guiding
   Educational Reform
time, 147–148
tool kit, 8–11
traditional teaching method, 3, 255
transitions, 95–96
trends, 262
Triangle of Integrated Learning.
      See Integrated Learning Triangle
verbal cues, 160
video learning, 107–108
virtual classes. *See* online education
virtual meetings, 262
virtual setting, 167
virtual tours, 158
virtual worlds, 174–175
visual image, 107
visual learning tools
   colors, 107
   flowcharts, 107
   graphs, 107

web
   classroom session, 4
   information access by, 57–58
   modules based on, 155
   NLN on, 40
   software for conferencing on, 160
web-based learning. *See* Online education
web conferencing software
   Blackboard, Collaborate Ultra, 160
   Elluminate, 160
   Zoom, 160
writing
   assignments, 78–79
   email, 85
   expectations of, 77
   objectives, 46–47
writing-to-learn, 79, 85